PE'

THE HANDBAG
Doctor

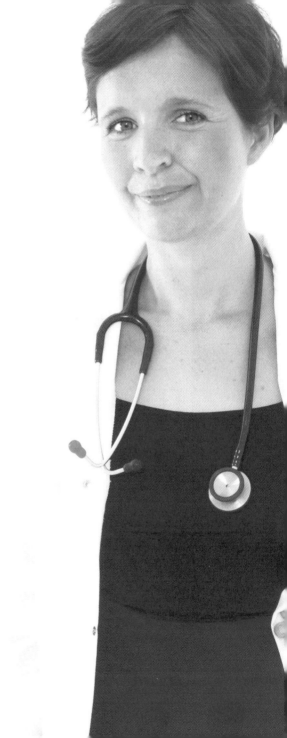

THE HANDBAG
Doctor

Sort your symptoms and
cure your ills: the indispensable
guide for women

Dr Pixie McKenna

Kyle Cathie Limited

For my favourite doctor, my Dad.

First published in Great Britain in 2010 by
Kyle Cathie Limited
23 Howland Street, London W1T 4AY
general.enquiries@kyle-cathie.com
www.kylecathie.com

10 9 8 7 6 5 4 3 2 1

ISBN 978-1-85626-934-6

Project editor: Jennifer Wheatley
Designer: Jane Humphrey
Illustrations: John Erwood
Copy editor: Carrie Walker
Editorial assistance: Catharine Robertson
and Elanor Clarke
Production: Gemma John

A Cataloguing In Publication record for this title
is available from the British Library.

Printed and bound by Great Britain by
Martins the Printers Ltd.

Disclaimer The contents of this book are for
information only and are intended to assist
readers in identifying symptoms and conditions
they may be experiencing. This book is not
intended to be a substitute for taking proper
medical advice and should not be relied upon
in this way. Always consult a qualified doctor
or health practitioner. The author and publisher
cannot accept responsibility for illness arising
out of the failure to seek medical advice
from a doctor.

Contents

INTRODUCTION

For me, my handbag doubles up as my head office. It's the hub of all my daily activity. You can find anything in there from a can of tuna to a pair of tights. When I need directions, I delve in to discover my A–Z; when I need resuscitation, I root out my lipstick. And I'm sure it's the same for you too. The handbag is not only a fashion accessory, but also a survival necessity. It's every woman's lifeboat.

This concept got me thinking – if the handbag was to be all things to all women, it needed its very own mini-medic, on call for all eventualities. And so The Handbag Doctor was born. A quick furrow round the handbag would release The Handbag Doctor, eager to dish out advice on various ailments – the good, the bad and the downright ugly!

My medical student days were spent sitting in lecture theatres absorbing information, only to regurgitate it again for end of term exams. But my patients have taught me far more than my six years at uni, that's for sure. The emotions of fear and shame are the two greatest barriers to both diagnosis and treatment, and that's one thing they don't teach you at medical school. I want The Handbag Doctor to help to allay people's unnecessary medical fears and anxieties, debunk myths and prompt every woman to seek medical advice however ashamed or scared she may be.

Many people are put off by medical jargon or the stuffiness and seemingly superior nature of my profession. I've tried hard to talk straight, so much so in fact that at times I had to stop myself putting some impolite words in! I've laid problems and symptoms out on the pages so that the information is plain to see, and I've given prompts about what you really should be discussing with and disclosing to your doctor. I want women to know when they should shout for help, but equally empower them to help themselves.

Many of us haven't got the time to see a doctor, and sometimes it seems the doctor doesn't even have the time to see us. But by consulting *The Handbag Doctor* as a symptom sorter, you can reassure yourself while you wait or reinforce the need to take time out and get checked. It's like triage by text. The general section at the beginning of the book is included with this in mind – a kind of hitlist of symptoms I see on a daily basis. It's for those odds and sods, those woolly problems that we all worry or wonder about. The list of course is not exhaustive, but it will hopefully guide you towards where to go next if you can identify yourself from the text.

I hope you benefit as much from reading *The Handbag Doctor* as I have from writing it. Although it's unlikely, you may be lucky enough never to have experienced any of the problems that appear in its 272 pages, but please don't shelve it on that basis. Let it lounge among the parking tickets, pens, take-away menus, cheque books and chewing gum in the microclimate of your 'must haves' because, like all the other seemingly superfluous stuff carried around in a handbag, it will, in time, be called on duty.

General symptoms

1

Not every symptom fits into a specific box. Here are some that make many women worry or simply wonder. If any relate to you, read on to find out where to go next for help.

Index

WHY DO I ACHE ALL OVER?

There are numerous causes for aches and pains in our joints, but the first thing someone usually asks their doctor is whether it could be arthritis. The type of arthritis we mean here is called osteoarthritis and is basically wear and tear on the joints, so it tends to come on in our mid-forties. It usually hits the bigger joints like the hips and knees.

You can't stop it, but you can improve the symptoms by keeping your weight down and remaining active. Glucosamine supplements have also been shown to help with pain in arthritic joints. They can be bought at the pharmacy and need to be taken in a dosage of 1500g a day. Arthritis often runs in families, so you may have a gran who had to get a new hip because her own wore out. But the fact of the matter is that we are all susceptible to arthritis whether or not grandma needed a new joint.

What about fibromyalgia?

With this, you hurt all over and tend to be very tired. You get generalised pain in your skeleton, with various trigger points that if touched produce sharp bursts of pain. Women – particularly middle-aged women – tend to suffer from this much more than men, and it is often seen in those with irritable bowel syndrome. It is often associated with problems sleeping, stiffness and a lack of clarity in memory and thinking – many call this the 'fibro-fog'.

Nobody really knows why fibromyalgia starts, and it can be extremely difficult to treat. Physiotherapy, exercise, acupuncture and analgesics (painkillers) are the mainstay of treatment, but it can be hit and miss. Many patients find it therapeutic to be part of a fibromyalgia support group as they often feel that doctors neither understand nor acknowledge the condition as there is no diagnostic test for it.

And rheumatoid arthritis?

This disease occurs when your body starts to reject your joints. We refer to this as an autoimmune disorder as you mount an immune response against yourself. It occurs most commonly in women, outnumbering men by three to one, and tends to come on in your forties. It can come on slowly or develop rapidly. The small joints of the hands and feet are typically affected and can become stiff, painful, swollen and inflamed. In one in five women the disease tends to be mild, while one in twenty have a very severe debilitating form. In its most severe form, you won't be able to do tasks like opening jars or doing up buttons. Rheumatoid arthritis is often accompanied by tiredness (see Tired all the time, page 13) The mainstay of treatment is preventing damage to the joints and easing the symptoms.

Could it be lupus?

This diagnosis needs to be in the mix if you feel tired and run down and have joint pain, stiffness and swelling. It is another autoimmune disease in which your immune system starts to attack your joints, blood vessels, skin, kidneys and other organs – we call it systemic lupus erythematosus (SLE) if it affects more than one body system. Ninety per cent of people who get this disease are women, and it mostly strikes between the ages of fifteen and forty-five.

As it can affect any organ in the body, its symptoms are varied, ranging from joint pain and tiredness to anaemia, kidney problems and skin rashes. Each case is different so lupus is often missed. If left unchecked, it can silently damage joints and vital organs like the kidneys, heart and brain and also result in recurrent miscarriage – missing this disease can have disastrous consequences. The difficulty is that there is no single blood test to diagnose it, so often there is more miss than hit. Ask your doctor to screen for autoantibodies – the antibodies that attack your system in autoimmune diseases – if you feel your body is letting you down and general blood results aren't coming up with any answers.

What should I say to my doctor?

All doctors regularly see patients with aches and pains. We tend to ask searching questions to work out why this is – we're not just being nosey; we have a real reason for asking. So tell your doctor about skin rashes, fevers, weight changes, night sweats, bowel symptoms, sleep problems, recent trips abroad, medicines you are taking, family history, joint swelling, urinary problems and energy levels. We need to know everything relevant to piece together the diagnosis.

The next step

Thyroid problems, diabetes, low levels of iron and vitamin B12 as well as other deficiencies (see the section on Diet and metabolism) can give you aches and pains. Standard blood profiles will be done to pick these up. We also check your blood for inflammation by doing what are called an ESR (erythrocyte sedimentation rate) and a CRP (C-reactive protein) blood test, as well as checking for rheumatoid factor and screening for autoantibodies. An infection screen for glandular fever and hepatitis (see the section on Infectious diseases) may also be considered, and urine tests may be sent off. Make an appointment to discuss the results with the doctor in a couple of weeks – this is much better than the 'no news is good news' approach.

Nothing sinister found?

Aches and pains can often be a symptom of low mood and generalised fatigue. Try some graduated exercise and adhere to a healthy diet. Consider the diagnosis of depression, and discuss this with your doctor or a friend if it could be relevant. Aches and pains are incredibly common during the menopause too. So don't despair that nothing has been found in blood tests; instead see it as a positive in that it signifies there is nothing untoward going on.

Tip ▌ *Joint aches and pains may be the first sign of a thyroid problem.*

I JUST CAN'T STOP SCRATCHING

Pruritis is the name given to any sensation that makes you want to scratch. Classic conditions such as eczema and dry skin cause this, as can psoriasis. Allergy and urticaria (aka hives) can make the skin feel it's on fire and heighten the desire to scratch.

Could it be an infection or an infestation?

Chicken pox is classically itchy, but you can rule this out if you've already had it. Scabies should be considered if the itch starts in the hands, with a rash that spreads onto the body. The peak time for scratching tends to be night-time. Scabies mites classically burrow and you might even witness them in your finger creases. Over-the-counter treatments are available at the pharmacist, and remember to boil-wash your bedclothes and treat your bed-fellows.

If it's not an allergy, infection, infestation or eczema, what's up?

If the cause isn't obvious or the condition is ongoing, go for a check-up as an underlying disorder can be found in 50 per cent of people with a generalised itch – kidney, liver or thyroid problems, lymphoma, iron deficiency or HIV. Tell the doctor if you are taking any medication, including vitamins or homeopathic treatments.

Itchy women

Two per cent of pregnant women have itching without a rash, which usually occurs in the last trimester. Many women also report the onset of itching when the menopause hits, compounded by the fact that skin is drying out.

What helps?

Most itching is worse at night so a sedating antihistamine helps then, with a non-drowsy antihistamine by day. The pharmacist can also make up a soothing mixture of menthol in aqueous cream. Dry skin obviously needs regular moisturisation. Use a light moisturiser as thick oily ointments can worsen the itch. It's imperative to have a check-up if you are suffering from itching in the absence of skin signs as this could be the first symptom of an underlying disease.

TIRED ALL THE TIME

This is an incredibly common reason for women to visit their doctor. Some look for reassurance that all's well; others strive to find answers for why they are run down. Doctors abbreviate this symptom to TATT, and I see at least one or two cases a day.

What's the cause?

Eighty per cent of women with this symptom don't have any serious underlying disease. The outcome of the consultation is that 'you are tired because you are tired'. This can be frustrating for everyone as it often results in the doctor being unable to help and the woman being no further forward in terms of a diagnosis.

What symptoms should I mention to my doctor to help the diagnosis?

Tell them about weight or mood change, sleep or appetite problems, night sweats, coughs, urinary symptoms, thirst, headache, recent foreign travel, changes in bowel habit, medications, drugs and alcohol, periods, work–life balance and stress.

Should I have any tests?

Yes, but first you should have a general examination. Your weight should be documented, and you should have a urine sample checked to rule out kidney disease and diabetes. Blood tests will be requested to check for anaemia, vitamin B12, white blood count, thyroid function, diabetes, blood chemistry and haematology, and markers of inflammation and infection. An infection screen may also be ordered specifically for glandular fever (see the Ears, nose and throat section) and hepatitis.

Common problems

Anaemia and vitamin B12 deficiency are common, and thyroid problems and diabetes can also crop up (see the section on Diet and metabolism). Serious problems such as leukaemia, lymphoma and kidney and liver disease will usually show on a blood test. If there is nothing unusual on this, you may be referred for a chest X-ray to look for TB or lymphoma. Depression is another common reason for TATT (see the section on Mental health) – if life isn't going well, your energy will be zapped.

Chronic fatigue syndrome

This has numerous names, from ME to post-viral fatigue syndrome and even yuppie flu. Some doctors doubt its existence, but it appears to occur in about three in every thousand people, with women suffering twice as often as men. The typical individual is in her thirties, and it's rare to see it in anyone over sixty. We don't know what causes it, but we see it more commonly as a consequence of glandular fever, in those with a history of depression and in high academic achievers. Having said that, it's not selective.

What are the symptoms? There will be a new onset of persistent tiredness, aches, pains and flu-like symptoms, a lack of any underlying medical condition, an inability to be refreshed by sleep yet wanting lots of it, total exhaustion after even minor physical activities such as shopping, not wanting to take part in social and professional activities, a lack of libido and an inability to concentrate. There is no specific diagnostic test, and it's more a question of ruling chronic fatigue 'in' rather than 'out'.

What's the treatment? It's very much trial and error. A gradual return to daily activities, graduated exercise and a healthy diet are advised. Some studies advocate using antiviral therapy over a period of six months. Antidepressant medication that has an activating effect, such as sertraline, can be considered as it serves to lift depression and improve energy. Cognitive-behavioural therapy can help people come to terms with their predicament.

Prognosis Fatigue lingers in about 50 per cent of people, and the longer you have it, the less likely you are to get fully better. Only a minority of clinics deal with this condition, but do try to get referred to one – it helps you get a better understanding of what's going on. Remember you're dealing with a condition for which there are no diagnostic tests and no specific treatments, so you must be open to trying things.

Tip *Don't put everything down to your chronic fatigue as it is possible to have co-existing pathologies. If new or unexplained symptoms arise, seek medical advice.*

PINS AND NEEDLES

Doctors term this numbness, pins and needles or tingling as 'paraesthesia'. It's usually temporary and felt in the hands and feet – for example after sitting awkwardly.

When should I go to the doctor?

Pins and needles tend to come and go. If it's a new symptom, a worsening trend or more frequent, visit your doctor. Do the same if it's associated with weakness or loss of function, you have problems passing urine or opening your bowels, or you have headaches, night sweats or tiredness.

What could be causing it?

Diabetes, alcohol and lack of vitamin B12 all have a role to play, as do some drugs, both prescription and recreational. Trapped nerves, thyroid problems and poor circulation can be involved, but numbness may be a sign of a problem in the nervous system.

What's the next step?

Your doctor will talk through your symptoms and do a full examination, including your reflexes and pain responses. Blood pressure and the eyes are also checked, and you will have blood and urine tests. If you still don't have an obvious diagnosis, a visit to the neurologist is likely. This will generally involve nerve and muscle tests and scans. It's true to say that, in young women, one of the first signs of multiple sclerosis can be – but most often isn't – pins and needles. Another less serious cause is panic attacks.

Lifestyle

Alcohol and bad diet may be implicated, so be prepared to change. Booze damages the nerve fibres in the same way as alcohol numbs pain. Vitamin B12 is found in meat and dairy produce but not vegetables, so a restrictive diet can cause deficiency.

Tip ▌ *Pins and needles occurring at the same time every day is probably related to physical activity.*

Myth ▌ *Pins and needles only occur in smokers. No, anyone can have them.*

I SWEAT LIKE A PIG

Excessive sweating is called hyperhydrosis. We wouldn't survive without sweating. It's the body's way of cooling itself down and is regulated by the sympathetic nervous system, the same wiring that speeds your heart up when you're scared. In 1 per cent of the population, this circuit is in overdrive and they sweat excessively.

So why is it happening to me?

There's often no reason, but it's well known with menopause, an overactive thyroid gland, certain drugs and anxiety. If you seem to sweat like a pig, see your doctor. You may need blood tests to rule out problems with your thyroid gland, blood count and hormones. You may need to stop certain medications – common culprits are antidepressants – or you may have an infection. Drenching night sweats may be due to tuberculosis (TB), lymphoma or malaria so see your doctor. If your blood tests and examination are clear, you are often defined as being sweaty just because you are. It's then you need to act, to stop the sweat yourself.

Why is sweat smelly?

Actually it isn't – it's the bacteria on the skin mixing with the sweat that make it reek. Some of our sweat glands are responsible for producing chemicals called pheromones, which produce a particular scent supposed to attract the opposite sex. But when the scent becomes a smell, you'll start to repel instead. We produce anywhere between one and five litres of sweat a day, and up to twelve litres if we trek across the desert. Our sweat glands really kick into action in response to our puberty hormones, which explains the distinct 'eau de teenager'.

How do I stop the sweat?

If there's no underlying problem, try aluminium chloride antiperspirants as these plug the pores and partially block the sweat glands. Although aluminium may sound toxic, it's safe for the sweat pores, and these antiperspirants are largely available without prescription.

Iontophoresis This works by passing electrical currents through the skin – and no, you can't get electrocuted, although you'll feel pins and needles. It's believed to stun the sweat glands into temporary submission. The treatment is available in hospitals, and you can buy your own machine. It usually takes four to seven treatments to stop sweating. All you do is place your hands and feet into baths filled with water and turn the current on. You usually need to do top-up treatments every so often.

Thoracic sympathectomy This surgical procedure is to be considered only after other methods have failed. A fine telescope is passed through the armpit under general anaesthetic and the lung is deflated. The telescope is then used to divide and remove the nerves responsible for sweating. The biggest problem is compensatory hyperhydrosis – medical speak for 'we fixed the sweating in that area, but it's come out somewhere else to compensate'. You may also suffer from gustatory hyperhydrosis, which is excessive sweating on eating, so surgery is not always the solution.

Botox We are all familiar with the magic properties of Botox for paralysing wrinkles, but it has another use in armpit sweating. Treatment involves about fifty injections into the armpit and needs to be repeated every four to six months. It acts by temporarily blocking the nerve that supplies the sweat gland.

Drugs Drugs that are used to dry up bladder problems are also used here. They can have side-effects like dry mouth and blurred vision but can provide a good stop-gap for people awaiting other procedures.

Simple measures Speak up about the problem and you'll find you're not alone. This condition isn't life or death, but if it is life-impacting, visit your doctor. Wear dark clothing and avoid man-made fibres. Keep your clothes loose and change them regularly as sweat dries in and no amount of cover-up will conceal it. Use antiperspirants and deodorants in combination – the latter only remove the smell – and make sure you wash well. Avoid excess alcohol, caffeine and spicy foods as they can all increase your sweat output.

IS FOUL BREATH MY FAULT?

Like it or not, at some point in your life you will suffer from bad breath – halitosis. People are often sent to their doctor or dentist by loved ones, friends, even their boss.

What are the culprits?

It's not rocket science to know that spices, garlic, cigarettes, alcohol and onions all make our breath smelly. So surely we should be all right if we can avoid them? Unfortunately, it's not that simple. Medical problems that can cause bad breath include sinus problems, tonsillitis, acid reflux, liver and kidney disease, mouth infections and some medications. The doctor may take a mouth swab or tongue scraping and send it to the lab to check for bacterial or other infections.

If the doctor has ruled out these problems, you are in the wrong surgery – get to the dentist. Poor oral hygiene is the most common cause of bad breath. It is important to brush for two full minutes twice a day. Time yourself – most of us do it for only thirty seconds. It's also necessary to brush your tongue, floss and use a mouthwash. Allocate five minutes to your teeth morning and night. That's a lot longer than you spend doing your mascara, so you'll need to build it into your routine.

And are your gums bleeding? You could have gingivitis – inflammation of the gums due to bacteria. It's the most common cause of tooth loss in the developed world. Smoking causes this too. Decayed teeth can be replaced by costly dental implants, but unless you ditch the smokes, these will succumb too.

Is it really important to floss? Yes, yes, yes. Imagine your mouth is like your rubbish bin: particles of food get trapped outside the bin-liner, so when you remove the rubbish bag, you don't always get all the rubbish. Food particles trapped between the teeth then get chewed up by bacteria in the mouth, and their waste products give that nice bad breath odour and gum disease.

LUMPS AND BUMPS ON MY SKIN

My doctor says I've got a dermatofibroma

This serious-sounding skin tumour is actually benign and incredibly common. Women outnumber men by four to one in the dermatofibroma stakes. It usually presents as a 'growth' on the lower leg. It feels like a lentil under the skin surface and can be skin-coloured, white or pinkish. It's little more than the skin's response to a previous injury such as an insect bite. They don't tend to grow or become bothersome so are best left well alone.

My doctor says I've got a lipoma

Lipomas are benign lumps of fat that grow under the skin and can vary from the size of a pea to a peach. They tend to feel firm yet smooth and crop up on the abdomen, neck, back and arms. Lipomas aren't dangerous and often occur in clusters. Unless they grow very big or are in an area that makes them unsightly, they don't need to be removed.

My doctor says I've got a sebaceous cyst

If you live long enough, you're likely to develop one of these. The twenties and thirties are the peak ages, and the cyst often arises as a painless bump under the skin. On close inspection, it may have a tiny pore, and if you dare to squeeze it, you'll be treated to a smelly cream-cheese substance. Cysts crop up on the face, neck, back, trunk and scalp. The problem is that they can increase in size and may become infected, so may need to be removed. The key tactic is to remove the entire cyst – any fragment left is likely to regrow. This procedure is easily done at the doctor's under local anaesthetic.

My doctor says I've got a ganglion

This is a little cyst that occurs next to the wrist. It's attached to either a bone or a tendon, so it moves freely under the skin. It's full of a gunky substance, like the inside of a jellyfish. There's usually no pain, but ladies are often keen to get rid of them as they look ugly. In times gone by, the ganglion was hit with the family Bible in an effort to

19

make it disappear. It's also possible to drain the fluid with a needle, but it usually fills up again in time. Surgery – thirty minutes under a local anaesthetic – generally provides a permanent cure.

My doctor says I have skin tags

Skin tags are very common and tend to occur in pressure areas like the collar, under the armpits or around the groin and buttock. They're just projections of skin popping up from the surface. They may be skin coloured or darker, and obese people are more susceptible. There's a 50/50 chance you have one or more, but don't fret as they aren't dangerous. Some patients 'self-doctor' and tie dental floss or thread around the stalk to cut off the blood supply. Tags can usually be cut off and cauterised (to stop the bleeding with heat) or frozen off as for warts. If the tag is very large, you may need an anaesthetic and a stitch. If you aren't bothered by the appearance and irritation, it's safe to leave them alone.

Things that go bump in the night

If you are worried about any lump or bump that has appeared on your skin, see your doctor. With a quick examination, they can usually reassure you of its origin. As you can see from the conditions above, most lumps and bumps are safe and need not concern us aside from the fact that they may look unsightly. Don't rush to have things removed if it's not necessary as the scar from the procedure is often more obvious than what was there in the first place (see the topic on Scars).

FEELING FAINT AND WOOZY

You'd be amazed how many people attend the doctor because they feel giddy or dizzy. Although for some of us that may be a normal state of mind, for others it may be a sign of an underlying problem. Women are twice as likely as men to have a full-blown faint, hence the need for gentlemen to give up their seats!

Gone out cold?

We have a lovely word for this: syncope. It is usually due to what's called a vasovagal attack. This simply means that a nerve called the vagus nerve gets overstimulated and brings about a rapid lowering of your heart rate and blood pressure. This causes you to fall to the floor – which restores your heart rate and blood flow, so no catastrophe. It generally occurs in times of prolonged standing, extreme heat, straining on the toilet, the sight of blood or having blood taken, fear or shock.

Tests There is often no need for testing, but if a faint isn't straightforward or attacks are recurrent, checks need to be made. Heart tests such as an electrocardiogram (ECG or EKG) can check the heart's rhythm as irregular beats can cause a collapse. Blood tests for diabetes or anaemia will also be ordered, as may blood pressure and heart monitoring over 24 hours. It is important to rule out problems with the heart, blood pressure, blood sugar level, circulation or blood count. By and large, no sinister cause is found in fit young women, and many are simply 'prone' to faints.

Feel faint but don't actually faint?

This is often due to dehydration or a low blood sugar, as well as low iron level, pregnancy or general fatigue. The difference here is that the brain has not taken over so you are in control and are able to sit, take a drink or get air.

Just dizzy or giddy?

This can happen for similar reasons but, depending on the frequency, it may require further checks. Dizziness and vertigo – a sensation of 'the spins' – may indicate a problem with the inner ear or blood supply to the brain. It may also be an effect of tablets such as beta-blockers taken for anxiety or high blood pressure. It is important to explain to the doctor exactly what you mean by dizziness – good balance depends on your brain, eyes and ears all working in sync.

Vertigo This gives rise to a sensation that you and the room are spinning. It can be due to a middle ear infection, problems with the balance receptors in the inner ear stimulated by sudden movement, or conditions such as Menière's disease in which fluid builds up in the middle ear, resulting in buzzing, vertigo and dizziness.

Working out the answers

We're all allowed a few faints in our lifetime, and at least half of us will keel over at some point. If you have a faint and it doesn't make sense, go and see your doctor. Although fainting is common, it's unusual to be a frequent fainter. In those over forty, fainting always warrants a visit to the doctor. As I said above, there are numerous reasons for hitting the deck. Most can be diagnosed at the doctor's by a simple examination and blood and urine tests. No further action is usually required, but that's no excuse for ignoring it. Missing something like an irregular heartbeat or a complication of a medication could prove catastrophic.

Tips *A danger time for fainting is prolonged standing on public transport the morning after the night before. The combination of low blood pressure, dehydration and a fast heart beat is a good mix for hitting the floor.*

Beware the hairdressers. Having your hair shampooed at the basin – especially if you are elderly – can provoke an attack because the tilt position may affect the blood flow to the head. So always sit for a few moments when you lift your head from the bowl.

RECURRENT MOUTH ULCERS

I'm being menaced by recurrent mouth ulcers

Mouth ulcers are a real menace. They are painful and prevent you eating properly, brushing your teeth or in some instances even talking. An ulcer occurs where there is any break in the surface membrane lining the gums, cheeks or tongue. It's painful because it results in exposure of the nerves that lie below the surface, so anything that touches it tweaks the nerves.

Aphthous ulcers

Twenty per cent of the population have recurrent ulcers at some point in their lives, women being affected more commonly than men. These ulcers tend to run in families and are kick-started by puberty. We call mouth ulcers aphthous ulcers if they have not occurred due to trauma, for example biting or burning your gum. In the majority of cases, the ulcers are tiny, generally less than 1cm in diameter. They are crater-shaped with a yellow–grey centre and a fiery red surround. They should disappear in about seven to ten days.

Why do I get ulcers?

Often, there is no reason for this, although stress is a major player, as is low immunity due to infection. There is also a genetic link whereby ulcers tend to run in families. So if both of your parents suffer, you unfortunately have a 90 per cent chance of mouth ulcer hell. Hormones can create them too, resulting in outbursts in the premenstrual period. Mouth ulcers can also occur due to nutritional deficiencies of, for example, iron, folic acid or vitamin B12 (see the section on Diet and metabolism).

Can I avoid ulcers?

Eat healthily and try to de-stress. Eliminate anything that is going to contribute to poor oral hygiene, such as smoking, and look after your teeth and gums well. Poorly fitting dentures and braces can contribute to ulcers, so see your dentist.

Can I treat them?

Yes, but if they are small, you often don't need to as they will disappear of their own accord. You can use a chlorhexidine-based mouthwash twice a day to prevent them becoming infected, and steroid lozenges or steroid gel can be used to stop the inflammation in the ulcer. Anaesthetic gels can also be rubbed on to the area they serve to cover the surface to protect it and kill the pain as well.

But what if they're really bad?

See your doctor as you may need to be treated with steroid tablets or mouthwashes and a course of antibiotics. This is, however, reserved for severe cases.

Should I have tests?

If you are having recurrent ulcers, yes, you should have basic blood tests that include iron, folic acid and vitamin B12 levels. Mouth ulcers are occasionally the first sign of a problem with the immune system, so your doctor will want to do a blood count and maybe even an HIV test. Diseases like coeliac disease and Crohn's disease that affect the gut can cause mouth ulcers too. If the diagnosis is in doubt, your doctor may in addition want to test for herpes as recurrent herpes infection can sometimes be the cause of recurrent ulcers (see the section on Infectious diseases). This is particularly important if you have any symptoms on your genitalia.

It is vitally important that any ulcer that persists for longer than four weeks is seen by a doctor or dentist – simple ulcers should be done and dusted after two to three weeks.

Tips   *If you stop smoking, your mouth ulcers will increase in frequency for a short period of time.*
      Act quickly on mouth ulcers and they'll heal more quickly. Have your treatment action pack at the ready just like you would for a cold sore.

COLD SORES

Why am I always breaking out in cold sores?

The very name sums up the misery of these beasts. They are generally caused by the type 1 herpes simplex virus (HSV); type 2 of this family of viruses causing genital herpes (see the section on Infectious diseases). Many of us come into contact with HSV, but not all are affected. Signs of the infection develop around the area where the herpes has entered the body, resulting in painful blisters on a red base. These generally tend to dry up and scab over, and can last seven to ten days. Cold sores, like genital herpes, can also cause systemic symptoms – doctors use this term to mean that you may have symptoms throughout the body such as fever, aches and pains, and enlarged glands.

Can you actually catch a cold sore?

Yes, and in fact most of us come into contact with the cold sore virus very early on in life as it's spread by kissing or by close contact with a cold sore. It's also possible to catch it from someone who doesn't have any signs of a cold sore but is shedding the virus from their skin or has it in their saliva.

Most of us acquire the initial infection as toddlers, and in fact 80 per cent of us have antibodies to it. Of those who have previously been infected, about one in five get recurrent cold sores. Once you have been exposed to the virus, it hides itself away in a nerve root and may reappear periodically.

What should I do?

Remember that cold sores are contagious so avoid close contact with people if you don't want to spread it. Remember too that although it's herpes simplex 2 that causes genital herpes, any active cold sores around the mouth can result in sores around the genitals if you engage in oral sex, and type 2 herpes can spread from the genitals to the mouth in the same way – so beware. Know what triggers your cold sore: stress, sunlight, infections, low immunity, fever, periods or even trauma to the skin can be a trigger. Often, however, there is no obvious trigger to awaken this sleeping virus.

As soon as a cold sore comes on, it needs treating. You can buy aciclovir (acyclovir) cream 5 per cent at the pharmacist, which you need to use five times a day for five days. The cream works best as soon as you feel the tingle.

What about recurrent sores?

You doctor can given you a course of tablets containing a form of aciclovir or another antiviral medicine. These can be taken in a low dose every day for three months or as a five-day course as soon as symptoms start. Try to minimise triggers by wearing sun block, eating well and de-stressing. If you seem to be getting more sores than usual, see your doctor as it could be the first sign your immune system is running low. And be sure of the diagnosis. If there is any doubt, ask your doctor to send a viral swab to the lab. It only takes ten seconds to take one, and it will confirm the diagnosis.

Will the cold sore spread?

Cold sores are contrary and tend to pitch up in the same position with each flare up, i.e. they have their 'patch'. However, it is important not to pick at the sore as you could potentially spread the virus to your eyes, resulting in inflammation there. It is also possible to spread the infection to your hands if you have cracked skin, causing blisters and infections on the fingers. Both of these need systemic treatment, i.e. pills.

Tip　*To avoid catching a cold sore, don't share lipsticks. And always wipe lipstick testers before using them, or test them on your hand.*

LOSS OF LIBIDO

Low libido is relatively common in ladies, but they often feel the doctor's surgery is not the place to discuss lack of 'mojo'. It's also important to differentiate between women who have always had a low libido and those who develop one. Many women suffer in silence, but as many as one in three sexually active women suffer from it at some point.

So what's up, doc?
There are numerous medical causes. A blood test to check for anaemia or thyroid problems is important, and underlying diseases like diabetes, heart problems or kidney disease are relevant. Some women experience a loss of libido in the menopause. Hormonal imbalance needs to be tested as excessive amounts of prolactin may be a cause, and low libido can be one of the first symptoms of depression.

Could I be causing it?
Excess alcohol consumption is a cause, so stick to your units. Recreational drugs such as cannabis can be a reason, as can prescribed drugs like tranquillisers, certain antidepressants and some contraceptives. Brands of contraceptive pill that have been around for decades – containing the progesterone hormones norethisterone or levonorgestrel – can typically hijack our libido.

Is it all in my head?
It's been said that the brain is the most important sexual organ, so anything going on in your head may cause your libido to lag. This can range from stress and anxiety to relationship issues, past sexual experiences and hang-ups.

What should I do?
The fact that there is no quick fix means women often just put up and shut up, but low libido for longer than three months deserves a visit to the doctor. Underlying causes can be ruled out, and if the cause doesn't seem physical, the psychological can be tackled. Psychosexual counsellors are excellent and often recommend you and your partner go back to basics and start 'courtship' again.

It's normal after a baby, right?

Fatigue is undoubtedly one thing to put the fire out, and there is nothing more tiring than a new baby. Add the hormonal fluxes and the physical consequences of delivery, and it's not surprising libido can be low. Mentally you are too tired, and physically you may be too sore. But this generally resolves. Although you may not be up for sex, don't lose the intimacy of a cuddle or a kiss. Keeping tactile is very therapeutic! However, remember that a low libido may also be a sign of postnatal depression, so chat to your midwife or doctor about how you're feeling.

The future

Some drugs, specifically testosterone and sildenafil (Viagra), have been used off licence for low libido. This means that although they have been prescribed, doctors don't have a licence to do so for this reason. The good news is that a drug in the pipeline – flibanserin – may help, so libido enhancement could be looking up for ladies.

'I have a headache'

Support from your partner is of paramount importance if this is going to be resolved, so talk about it – shying away results in perfunctory sex and makes the problem worse. Remember that our sexual brain works on the premise of libido, then arousal and finally orgasm. Without step 1, steps 2 and 3 are often unobtainable. It's important to make sure your mate realises that the female libido has been likened to damp wood – frustrating to ignite, but persist and you'll start a fire!

Tips

Fatigue floors your libido so get some sleep.

Pelvic floor exercises (see the topic on Bladder control) can improve your sex life, so get squeezing. And although discussions on prolapse and post-pregnancy perineums may not seem up your street, check out the advice available.

Myth

Menopause zaps the libido. Not necessarily – many women feel sexually liberated and enjoy an even better sex life.

FLATULENCE

One wonders why a lady would need to know anything about this; surely it's the domain of men! Sorry, girls, but we do actually pass wind up to thirteen times a day and can be responsible for between 500ml and two litres of gas being let out into the atmosphere. There is, in fact, no scientific difference between men and women in terms of flatus.

What makes us pass flatus?

Swallowing air is one cause, so smoking, chewing gum and not chewing your food properly could be a problem. Certain foods make us more windy, for example carbohydrates, vegetables such as beans, cabbage, broccoli and Brussels sprouts, lentils and fruit such as prunes. Medical conditions can also be an issue:

▌ Constipation

▌ Irritable bowel syndrome and coeliac disease

▌ Lactose intolerance, or an inability to break down the sorbitol in diet drinks or the fructose found in fruits

▌ Anything that alters the gut bacteria, for example diarrhoea or antibiotics.

The gas we produce when the bacteria have broken down our food is a mixture of nitrogen, methane, hydrogen, oxygen and hydrogen sulphide, and it's the latter that smells. Foods rich in sulphur, such as cauliflower, eggs and meat, will make wind smellier. Some vegetables, such as green beans, contain a type of carbohydrate that is indigestible for humans. Sorbitol, often found in chewing gum and artificial sweeteners, is also indigestible and will contribute to wind.

Diagnosis As you can probably guess, there's no diagnostic test for this.

How you can help yourself

If you are a windy woman, exercise, as it stimulates digestion. Watch your diet – avoid carbohydrates, sweeteners or anything that makes you more flatulent. Go to the doctor if you have also had any weight loss, altered bowel function or new symptoms.

IS MY LIFESTYLE DAMAGING MY LIVER?

Your liver sits on the right of your body under your rib cage. You can't see it or feel it on the outside, but unbeknown to you, it's working hard on the inside. Ask people what role the liver plays and most will mention alcohol. Yes, it does act to process alcohol, but it also has over six hundred other functions so understandably it gets irritated when it becomes overrun with booze.

What does the liver do?

The liver is like a chemical processing factory, breaking substances down, processing them, storing them and producing new products every second of the day. We cannot live without it. Like all factories it will do overtime when needed, but constant pressure on the workforce and resources, such as from a large amount of alcohol, ultimately means that the production line suffers and processes start to break down.

What's safe?

Women should not drink more than fourteen units per week and more than three per day. We are often 'woolly' about what we consider to be a unit: a large glass of Pinot Grigio in a hotel bar may mean you tot up three units in one go, so beware of your measures. It is fairly easy for your doctor to see whether you liver is happy by checking your liver function tests. A high level of a liver enzyme known as gamma-GT is a very sensitive indicator of alcohol consumption, so although you may be telling your doctor you are abstemious, your blood will tell a different story. As a rule of thumb, try to stick within safe guidelines and make sure you give your liver a rest by having regular weekly alcohol-free days, ideally two in every seven.

Problems that develop

If you drink more than your liver can handle, fat will be deposited around it. If you keep on drinking, your liver will become inflamed – hepatitis. Ignore this sign to stop and there is a 10–20 per cent chance that you will develop cirrhosis of the liver. There is no going back from this condition as the liver cells die and only a transplant can save you. In the UK alone, around four hundred people die of liver disease each day.

Women and alcohol

Overweight women who drink too much are far more susceptible to liver disease, and one in three women drink more than the safe limits. Women also like to binge – as medics, we define this as twice our daily units. So ladies, six units, or put practically two large glasses of wine at lunchtime, qualifies as a binge. Alcohol has other specific dangers for women, such as increasing the risk of cancers such as breast cancer, causing problems with fertility and leading to depression. In addition, one in six women would admit to having had unprotected sex after a boozy binge.

Know your units

We often 'guesstimate' our units and, let's be fair, underestimate them. So here's how to work it out:

Strength × Volume ÷ 1000 = Number of units

11.5% Pinot Grigio white wine × 250ml size glass ÷ 1000 =
11. 5 × 250 ÷ 1000 = 2.875 units

The strength is the 'ABV' (alcohol by volume), which will written be on the side of the bottle. The volume is the size of the glass. Multiply them together and divide by 1000 and you get your units. Adding up the sum of what you have drunk at the end of the night can be as scary as looking into your wallet!

THE CAGE QUESTIONNAIRE

If you answer yes to two or more of these questions it is considered clinically significant.	Have you ever felt you should **C**ut down on your drinking?	Yes/No
	Have people **A**nnoyed you by criticising your drinking?	Yes/No
	Have you ever felt bad or **G**uilty about your drinking?	Yes/No
	Have you ever had a drink first thing in the morning to steady your nerves or to get rid of a hangover (**E**ye opener)?	Yes/No

Gynaecology

2

Like it or not, our gynaecological kit can sometimes cause mischief, so here are the problems that are most likely to bother you and how to get them treated.

THE FEMALE REPRODUCTIVE ORGANS

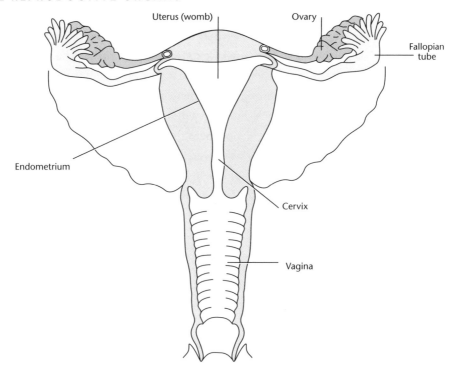

Uterus (womb)

Ovary

Fallopian tube

Endometrium

Cervix

Vagina

HEAVY PERIODS

Menorrhagia is the medical jargon for heavy periods. A loss of 80ml or more of blood over the menstrual period is defined as menorrhagia – that's the amount that would fill a small wine glass. The average woman loses about half this amount, and although many of us report heavy periods, only about one in ten of us are losing more than 80ml of blood per cycle. Let's be fair though, it is incredibly hard to quantify, so if your periods are too heavy for you, seek help. As a rule, your flow is probably too heavy if you have to use pads and tampons at the same time, if you experience clots or flooding, and if pale clothing is a 'no no'. If the heaviness of your flow is affecting you personally or professionally, that's the time to shout for help.

What could the problem be?

Here we go again in terms of doctors not having the answers – in 50 per cent of cases we simply don't know. If we truly don't know why, we refer to it as dysfunctional uterine bleeding. The causes we *can* identify include the following:

▌ Fibroids – muscular growths in the wall of the womb that grow in response to the female hormone oestrogen. They tend to result in heavy periods.

▌ Polyps in the cervix –little fleshy growths that appear at the opening of the cervix and can bleed heavily during menstruation. Like fibroids, they are benign.

▌ Pelvic inflammatory disease – an infection in the reproductive tract. It can also cause heavy bleeding and can be due to an infection such as Chlamydia.

▌ Having the copper coil for contraception.

▌ Cancer of the lining of the womb may be a cause in women over forty.

▌ Endometriosis, blood clotting disorders and thyroid problems.

What should I do?

Fill in a menstrual diary. This gives the doctor a really good picture of how much blood you are losing and how it is affecting you, because when you talk about it, its impact is often not as clear.

Book an appointment when you are mid-cycle, otherwise you doctor will not be able to fully examine you. And remember to tell the doctor about any problems with your bowels or bladder. It is also important to relate any symptoms of discharge, painful sex or bloatedness. Volunteer the information if you aren't asked.

Investigations

Your doctor will examine your tummy to check if there is anything to feel. This is often followed by a pelvic examination to feel for fibroids and an examination to look at your cervix. You may have some swab tests to check for infections and a blood test to check your iron levels, clotting factors and thyroid gland function.

If your doctor is happy with the results of these but still believes there might be a problem, you will probably be referred for a scan. This will check for fibroids, look at your ovaries and assess the thickness of the lining of the womb. It is generally done by placing a probe into the vagina so again needs to be timed around mid-cycle.

Enough tests; what's next?

If it has been established that you have dysfunctional uterine bleeding, you have several options, most of which are available on prescription. If you need contraception, the oral contraceptive pill is an option as it has the added benefit of making your periods lighter and shorter. The progesterone hormone called norethisterone, which is also found in the mini-pill, can be given three times a day from day 5 to day 26 of your menstrual cycle and works to lessen blood flow. It does not, however, act as a contraceptive, so beware and take other precautions.

A MENSTRUAL DIARY

Month

Day	1	2	3	4	5	6	7	8	9	10	11	12	13	14	15	16	17	18	19	20	21	22	23	24	25	26	27	28	29	30	31
Menstrual flow (see box 1)																															
Pain level (see box 2)																															

Month

Day	1	2	3	4	5	6	7	8	9	10	11	12	13	14	15	16	17	18	19	20	21	22	23	24	25	26	27	28	29	30	31
Menstrual flow (see box 1)																															
Pain level (see box 2)																															

Month

Day	1	2	3	4	5	6	7	8	9	10	11	12	13	14	15	16	17	18	19	20	21	22	23	24	25	26	27	28	29	30	31
Menstrual flow (see box 1)																															
Pain level (see box 2)																															

Menstrual flow
+++ Heavy *Needing sanitary towels as well as tampons. Large clots and/ or flooding (blood staining clothes or bedding).*
++ Moderate *Regular changing of towels or tampons. No social inconvenience.*
+ Light *Needing some protection to prevent staining of underwear.*
S Spotting *Very light loss staining underwear.*

Pain level *(Fill in if in any pain)*
+++ Severe *Requiring painkillers. Not able to do normal activities.*
++ Moderate *Needing mild painkillers. But able to carry on normal activities.*
+ Mild *But not needing painkillers.*

If you don't want hormones, you can use mefenamic acid, which blocks the prostaglandin chemicals that stimulate bleeding. This can cut blood loss by as much as 50 per cent. The beauty is that it's also a painkiller so works for period pain too. It's not suitable for those who cannot take anti-inflammatories and if you have some types of asthma or a stomach ulcer. You can also opt for tranexamic acid. This helps blood to clot and may cut bleeding by half.

If you don't want to take tablets, the coil containing the levonorgestrel is ideal. It works fantastically well in decreasing blood flow and doubles up as a very reliable contraceptive. It will usually leave you with a day's light flow a month, but for some women, periods may disappear altogether. This coil is safe and can be left in for five years – your doctor or family planning clinic can insert one for you.

A trip to the gynaecologist?

If you're bleeding heavily, are over forty-five or treatment isn't helping, you're likely to be referred to a gynaecologist, who may do a scan and take a sample of the womb lining to check for anything cancerous. Polyps or fibroids will be removed, the former usually in outpatients, the latter under general anaesthetic.

Will I need a hysterectomy?

Not necessarily. If you have heavy periods and have completed your family, you may be suitable for endometrial ablation, which involves burning, lasering or even microwaving the lining of the womb. Seventy per cent of women report lighter periods six months after the procedure, and some have no periods whatsoever. Hysterectomy may be necessary in women who have other problems such as fibroids, or if other treatments are unsuitable or have failed. A hysterectomy will keep you in hospital for days whereas an endometrial ablation can be done as a day case. You could be back at work one week after an ablation, but it will be at least four to six weeks after a hysterectomy.

The bottom line

The physical practicalities of a haemorrhage once a month can be horrific in terms of day-to-day activities. There is also a physiological cost in terms of anaemia. So seek help if you feel your flow is too heavy.

FIBROIDS

One in three of us women will have fibroids at some point, but we usually won't have symptoms. Fibroids generally only cause mischief when they enlarge, and can be as small as a pencil tip or large as a melon. They feed on our female hormone, oestrogen, so they grow bigger in pregnancy and on the Pill, and shrink in the menopause.

How would I know if I had a fibroid?

Heavy periods are common. Feeling bloated or having a tummy that looks like it's pregnant can be a sign. You may also constantly feel pressure on your bladder and need to go the toilet, and you may feel constipated. The doctor may be able to feel them on an internal examination, and an ultrasound scan will show them up.

Who gets them? Women in their thirties and forties, women who are overweight and women with a family history of fibroids. Afro-Caribbean women are three times more likely to get them.

Can they be removed? Medicine can't cure fibroids, but it can shrink them. Drugs called gonadotropin releasing hormone analogues can do this if your doctor plans to remove the fibroids by surgery as it makes the surgery easier. These drugs cause a mini-menopause and lower oestrogen levels. Because of the side-effects, such as hot flushes and osteoporosis, they are not for long-term use.

Uterine artery embolisation is a new treatment with uncertain long-term results. It involves blocking the blood supply to the fibroid, causing it to shrink, and gives about two thirds of women relief. Myomectomy – surgical removal – can be done by open surgery, through either the vagina or abdomen, or via a telescope into your abdomen.

What should I be on the look out for?

Bloatedness, heavy periods and pressure to go the toilet are common. It is also important to be aware that fibroids can cause problems in pregnancy or make it difficult to fall pregnant depending on where in the womb they are. Your doctor will send you for a scan if there are any doubts.

37

ENDOMETRIOSIS

Endo what? In the UK, about 2 million women are affected by it – that approximates to the population of Paris. But although you may have heard of it because it's common, can you define what it is?

What is it and why does it happen?

It occurs when patches of endometrium – womb tissue – find themselves outside the womb. These patches occur in the tubes, ovaries, vagina and rectum, even the lungs. This tissue breaks down and bleeds with each menstrual cycle, just as womb tissue does, and this is what causes the problem. So how does that happen? Well, it may be the twenty-first century but science isn't really sure. Many theories have been put forward, but none is fact.

If it's that common, could I have it?

Yes, you could, if you have any of the following symptoms: painful periods, heavy periods, pain with sex, back pain or diarrhoea with periods, infertility or irregular bleeding.

Can the doctor diagnose it with a blood test?

No, it's diagnosed under anaesthetic by a gynaecologist with a telescope (called a laparoscope) who looks into the pelvis and actually sees the endometriosis.

Treatment Unfortunately, we can't cure endometriosis. However, treating the pain with anti-inflammatories generally helps. Use medication such as ibuprofen or naproxen as these work better than paracetamol. Mefenamic acid is available on prescription and acts on the chemicals that cause period pain. It should be taken throughout your period, but a clever trick is to start it a couple of days before your period is due.

Hormone treatment also works well. The combined oral contraceptive pill can help make cycles shorter, lighter and less painful; it's a combination of the hormones oestrogen and progesterone taken to prevent ovulation. Other hormone preparations work by mimicking a menopause, so they aren't without side-effects, for example weight gain, acne, mood problems and sometimes excess hair growth. The 'anti-progestogens' work by inhibiting ovulation and also shrinking the womb tissue, but as progesterone is the hormone that causes premenstrual syndrome, this treatment can have similar effects.

Surgery is another option. Patches of endometriosis can be burned off by the surgeon when looking inside you with the laparoscope. Endometriosis also causes adhesions – it's just like throwing chewing gum into your pelvis; it makes things stick together. These adhesions can also be divided at the time of your laparoscopy.

When endometriosis is severe and conservative surgical and medical management have failed, hysterectomy may be the final option. We call this radical surgery because it is. It's a major surgical procedure and not without complication. It would only ever be offered to women who have completed their families and those whose case is so life-impacting that there is no other option. You would never be asked to make this decision abruptly, and with good conservative management you will hopefully never need to contemplate it.

Problems with endometriosis

Here's a condition that's very common, we aren't sure what causes it, we can't cure it, yet it can give rise to major complications. One in four women who find it difficult to fall pregnant have endometriosis. Old textbooks also state that pregnancy is helpful in reducing the symptoms of endometriosis, but of course falling pregnant proves difficult. The condition is often brushed aside as 'bad periods', and you only realise it is a problem when falling pregnant also becomes a problem.

If your periods are dire and you decide to see the doctor, take a diary of symptoms, a tally of pads and tampons used and days off work, a list of things you do to alleviate your symptoms and a description of how it affects you and those around you. This will help you and your doctor to devise a management plan together.

Tips ▌ *Endometriosis can sometimes mimic the symptoms of irritable bowel syndrome, so beware.*
▌ *Don't wait years to tackle problem periods as you could end up having difficulty falling pregnant.*

WHEN SEX HURTS

Doctors call this dyspareunia, and women often simply put up with it. There is a myriad of causes, the clue often lying in the history rather than the physical examination. But it can't be fixed if you don't ask for help.

What could be wrong if it's painful deep inside?

If you are experiencing deep dyspareunia (i.e. when he is inside), you may have a fibroid, an infection, a problem with your ovaries, a problem with your cervix or adhesions from previous surgery. You will usually have other symptoms though, such as heavy or painful periods, discharge, discomfort, irregular bleeding, bloating or bladder symptoms.

What if intercourse is painful going in?

Lack of lubrication can be a problem, often due to a failure to be aroused, as can vaginal dryness around the menopause. Infections such as thrush (candida), herpes, warts or Trichomonas can all cause pain on entry. Some ladies get a dermatitis on the outside due to bubble baths, spermicides or latex condoms, resulting in the exterior being inflamed and sore. Episiotomy scars can give rise to pain too.

What else could it be?

When these causes have been excluded, you need to explore other factors. Vaginismus is a condition where the muscles of the vagina go into spasm, and it can result in both deep and superficial pain. It is often so painful the woman is unable to have full intercourse or even a smear test. There may be no reason, but a history of one of the problems outlined above can set up a vicious cycle of spasm as the woman anticipates pain and shuts down. There may have been a bad sexual experience or assault in the past, and as soon as the penis approaches the vagina, it simply tightens up.

Vulvodynia is a condition in which the external female genital organs are hypersensitive –even touching them triggers impulses of pain. Nobody really knows why this happens, but any of the causes that result in superficial pain may contribute.

How to get help

Only one in every four women who have this problem discuss it with their doctor. Like you, doctors may be uncomfortable talking about sex. But to get a full history of dyspareunia, you need to be prepared to tell all. Don't book a hurried consultation with a doctor you don't get on with, as it will end in disaster. You will need to go mid-cycle as you are likely to need an examination. And remember that if you don't explore the causes, it may never go away.

Can you fix it?

All the physical problems mentioned above can be managed via your family doctor. If you are suffering from vaginismus, you are likely to be helped greatly by a psychosexual counsellor who will train you on the use of vaginal dilators. These range in size, and you gradually insert them twice a day for ten or fifteen minutes each. When you can use the smallest trainer without difficulty, you graduate to the next. This is slow process, so be patient.

Your psychosexual counsellor will also coach you through rediscovering your sexual relationship with your partner. This is likely to involve several stages, starting with courtship, so you may find a sex ban is imposed as you get back to basics. The aim is to learn how to make sex more enjoyable, not just for your partner but importantly for yourself.

Vulvodynia can often be helped by drugs that block pain, for example amitriptyline. Anaesthetic gels can be used for short-term management. Psychosexual counselling can also be helpful here to help you work through the relationship difficulties associated with this condition. Wearing cotton underwear, not using scented soaps and avoiding prolonged sitting, cycling or horse-riding can also help.

Tip   *IBS may be making sex sore.*

GENITAL WARTS

There are two words to describe genital warts: rampant and permanent. They are the most common sexually transmitted infection, and are caused by the human papilloma virus (HPV). This is essentially the wart virus and there are over a hundred types, so there are plenty out there to catch. These HPV viruses cause not just genital warts, but also verrucas and other warts. Genital warts are spread though sexual as well as skin-to-skin contact, so condoms will not completely protect you. If you come into contact with the virus, the warts usually appear two to four weeks later, although it can take months.

Where do they crop up?

Warts tend to grow on the inner lips, the opening of the vagina and inside it. They can also appear on the cervix, anus or perineum (the bit between your front and back bottom!). In men, they tend to be visible on the penis, scrotum and anus; they can also hide under the foreskin. They can also be found in the groin in both sexes. Oral sex with an infected person can result in them cropping up in the mouth and sometimes on the face. Beware, just because you can't see any warts, it doesn't mean there isn't a wart virus infection – there is an incubation period between the time you contract the virus and the time the warts appear.

What do they look like?

They can be raised and look like a cauliflower, or flat or small. They occur in clusters or on their own and are skin-coloured. Some are thin and wispy, whereas others grow on stalks. Generally, they aren't sore, but they can be itchy or irritating.

How are they diagnosed?

Usually by examination – they have a very distinct appearance to a doctor. Many patients unfortunately do not know what they are and have them for years before seeking medical attention. Warts around the anus are commonly mistaken for piles.

Treatment There are two different types of prescription treatment. One contains podophyllin, which chemically burns the wart off. You apply it at home twice daily, three times a week for four weeks. The other treatment attacks the immune system and is applied twice daily for twelve weeks.

Warts can also be frozen off or painted with high-strength caustic podophyllin. Occasionally, they are cut out or treated with laser. Whatever treatment you opt for, you will never entirely get rid of the wart virus – the propensity for warts to make a comeback is always there.

Problem Types HPV16 and HPV18 have been proven to cause abnormal cells on the cervix, which can result in cervical cancer – so genital warts not only cause embarrassment, but also have the potential to cause serious health problems. By the time most girls are twenty-six there is at least a 50/50 chance that they have come into contact with the wart virus.

This is serious stuff, ladies. If you have had warts, make sure you are up to date with your cervical smear. Ask too to be tested for the dangerous forms of HPV. The up-and-coming teens are now being vaccinated against these virus types via the cervical cancer vaccination programme. This means they will be immune to the dangerous types of wart virus before they come into contact with them.

Who gave the warts to whom?

The chain of evidence is always difficult. If you have sex with someone with warts, you may develop warts between two weeks and two months later. There is also a possibility that the warts may not appear for years, or they may never appear. Sometimes a partner had warts many years ago and the warts have come back at a time of stress or when the person is run down. The bottom line is that the appearance of warts does not always signify infidelity. What it does signify, however, is that treatment is warranted and that cervical smears need to be kept up to date.

THRUSH

Have you ever met anyone called Candida? Well, that's the other name for thrush! Funnily enough, thrush is also the name given to a bacterial infection that can occur in a horse's hoof. I'm sure most of us haven't suffered from that, but three quarters of us will have a bout of thrush (candidiasis) at some point in our lives. It is incredibly common.

What are the symptoms?
It's the onset of itch which usually signals that the thrush has landed. This can be accompanied by irritation and discomfort externally that can sometimes make it uncomfortable to pass water. Discharge is another symptom, and this is generally creamy white. Thrush can also make sex painful, both when going in and deep inside.

Why does it happen?
Deep inside the vagina, bacteria and yeast live side by side, but sometimes the yeast tries to take over. It multiplies in numbers and this overgrowth is what causes the symptoms of thrush to occur. So rather than yeast itself being the problem, it's the amount of it. The things that trigger this include antibiotics, stress, recurrent sexual activity, periods, pregnancy and wearing tight clothing. Using douches or perfumed bubble baths doesn't help either. And some contraceptive pill-takers suffer from it.

What should I do?
If you think you may have thrush, seek advice from your pharmacist as most treatments are available over the counter. Remember that although you may have symptoms outside the vagina, you will also need to hit the thrush internally. This is done by using a cream on the outside, and then inserting a cream or tablet via an applicator into the vagina. A word of warning though: if you are inserting vaginal creams, do it at night as they can be messy and seep out onto your underwear. A one-off pill is also available; this is taken by mouth and serves to strike out thrush both inside and out. And beware – creams and pessaries may damage condoms.

How can I help prevent thrush?

Avoid the skinny jeans and the tight synthetic fibre underwear, girls. They are the enemy in the thrush stakes. Don't linger in a bubble bath or use perfumed gels and soaps. And change your tampons on a regular basis. Like all fungus, thrush flourishes in a moist, dark, warm environment, so make sure you wash and dry yourself thoroughly, especially after exercise.

Recurrent thrush

First things first – you need to check that it really is thrush. Go and see your doctor and have a swab as this could be a sexually transmitted infection. If you are feeling tired and run down, your doctor might suggest a blood glucose test for diabetes or a blood count to check your immune system, as it may be the first sign of another illness. If you definitely have recurrent thrush, your doctor may prescribe a tablet to be taken every day for a week or a tablet to be taken once a month for six months. Your partner will only need to be treated if they have symptoms.

What's the alternative?

Many women use natural yoghurt on tampons that they insert for seven nights. If you do decide to follow this alternative option, make sure it is unsweetened plain live yoghurt as anything else may encourage yeast growth. You might find it easier to eat it though – both methods are found to ease symptoms but are not necessarily a cure. Garlic and tea tree oil can also be used.

Tip | *Look for thrush in the mouth; it causes white patches on the tongue. If you don't treat it up top, it may never resolve down below.*

Pitfall | *All that discharges is not thrush – it might be time for a test for a sexually transmitted infection.*

VAGINAL DISCHARGE

Fishy, creamy, frothy… there are a multitude of descriptions for discharge. Discharge does not always indicate sexually transmitted disease, so don't despair. It is normal to have some form of discharge varying in consistency through the menstrual cycle. Normal physiological discharge varies throughout the cycle, being clear and wet before ovulation and then thick and sticky afterwards. Some people observe their cervical mucus to see when they are most fertile. The normal discharge is generally either clear or whitish, it doesn't smell and it doesn't irritate. Discharge that deviates from the norm, smells or looks offensive and is associated with other symptoms needs checking.

Thrush

Creamy white discharge with associated itch and irritation is usually due to thrush (candidiasis), and three out of every four of us will get thrush at some point. Thrush isn't sexually transmitted and is easily treated. We see it more frequently in people with diabetes, those on antibiotics and those with a poor immune system. However, most people who suffer from thrush are perfectly healthy. It's simple to treat with over-the-counter medications and creams. If it's recurrent, your doctor may put you on a week-long course of anti-thrush tablets.

Bacterial vaginosis

A fishy-smelling watery discharge without itch or irritation is due to bacterial vaginosis. Fifty per cent of those who have it don't know they do, and it generally goes unnoticed in women who are not pregnant. It's not sexually transmitted, but it can cause pain during intercourse. It can, however, be dangerous in pregnancy as it can cause premature labour and membrane rupture.

Retained tampon

It never ceases to amaze me how common this is. If you forget to remove a tampon, it will result in a foul-smelling, often blood-stained discharge. By foul-smelling, I really do mean foul! A tampon left in for over a week is so malodorous it can make you retch. It's usually easy for the doctor to make the diagnosis by doing an internal examination and then removing the offending item with forceps. It generally tends to be impossible for women to remove the tampon themselves as it is too far inside. If in any doubt, see your doctor, as leaving it there can result in serious infection.

Problems with the cervix

Polyps can grow inside the cervix or the lips of the cervix can become inflamed, resulting in discharge, bleeding in between periods and painful sex. Persistent vaginal discharge is sometimes the first sign of a cervical cancer.

Allergic reactions

Allergy to latex and semen can cause problems, as can douching. This can result in discharge and irritation.

Sexually transmitted infections

Chlamydia can cause a pussey discharge and is usually associated with painful sex or urinary symptoms. Gonorrhea can give rise to a green discharge, bleeding in between periods and pain passing urine. *Trichomonas vaginalis* can cause yellow discharge, itching and irritation externally.

What should I do?

See your doctor if you have any of the following: increased discharge, blood-stained, green or offensive discharge, urinary symptoms or pelvic pain, recurrent 'thrush', or at least what you think is thrush, or external itching and irritation.

What will happen?

The doctor will ask you lots of specific questions about the discharge, its associated symptoms and your sexual activity. Answer the questions honestly, otherwise it may be impossible to get to the bottom of it. The doctor will then examine you internally (as for a smear test), take swabs of the discharge and probably send off a urine test as well. The lab will then confirm the cause. So if you've got a discharge, no matter how embarrassed you are, get to the doctor and get a diagnosis.

Tip ▮ *Don't self-diagnose yourself as having recurrent thrush – see the doctor. It could be a sign of diabetes, or you could actually have a sexually transmitted infection.*

CONTRACEPTION – ARE YOU COVERED?

There are over a dozen different choices, and you need to make the right one. However barren you think you are, you need cover unless you are keen on having a baby – even up to one year after your periods have stopped.

So what about the pill?

The combined pill contains two hormones – oestrogen and progesterone. Oestrogen is our gender hormone. Progesterone is made during the second half of our menstrual cycle and is responsible for PMS. Its peak results in symptoms of acne, bloating and irritability. These two hormones are combined in one tiny pill and stop us from falling pregnant by halting our ovaries. You take the pill every day for twenty-one consecutive days and then have a break for seven days, during which you have a period. Generally, taking the pill makes your periods lighter, shorter and less painful. If you take it as instructed, it's 99 per cent effective. The added bonus is that it protects against ovarian cancer.

Doesn't it cause clots? Yes, but for every ten thousand women taking it for a year, fewer than three will suffer a clot. You're less likely to get a clot – legs or lungs – than if you were pregnant. If you're overweight, immobile, a smoker or have high blood pressure, you're at higher risk, and women over thirty-five who smoke are never prescribed the combined pill. Migraine sufferers who have attacks lasting three days, get recurrent attacks or have symptoms such as blurred vision should not take it as it can increase the risk of stroke. Never forget to tell any doctor you are on the pill, especially if you are going for surgery as it increases your risk of clots.

Are there any other problems? Breast discomfort and enlargement, acne, low mood, weight gain, thrush, reduced libido, nausea, migraine, headache and fluid retention can all occur. Because the pill shuts off ovulation, some women find their periods do not return for a while after stopping it. If this goes on longer than six months, see your doctor. When you first start the pill, you may experience breakthrough bleeding or spotting for the first three months – if it goes on for longer than this, it needs checking.

Check-ups You doctor will want to see you every six months to monitor your blood pressure. If you don't like your pill, shout – there are many available and what suits your friend may be your personal foe. Remember that you won't be immune to sexually transmitted infections: you need regular checks and smears. The policy of 'double-wrapping' by using condoms as well is not only preventative, but also helps ward off sexually transmitted infections.

The mini-pill

This came onto the market for those unsuitable for the combined pill. It contains only one ingredient – progesterone. This works by affecting the cervical mucus to make it difficult for sperm to get in, and also thins the womb lining, making implantation less likely. It can be 99 per cent effective if taken correctly. Unlike the combined pill, it is taken every day without a withdrawal break. It is the ideal choice for women over the age of thirty-five who smoke but still want to take a pill. The problem is that it needs to be taken at the same time every day, with only a three-hour window of error. The good news is there is now a new mini-pill in the UK – Cerazette – that prevents ovulation as well and has a twelve-hour window. The side-effects of the mini-pill are acne, bloatedness, breast pain, erratic bleeding or absence of periods.

What about contraceptive injections or implants?

This type of contraception, which contains progesterone, is injected every twelve weeks into the buttock or administered as a tiny implant under the skin of the upper arm. The implant lasts for three years. Its safety is similar to the progesterone-containing mini-pill, but it's far more effective – over 99 per cent. It stops ovulation and alters the cervical mucus so that pregnancy is less likely.

Like the mini-pill, you can experience the PMS-like side-effects of progesterone. Most women who stop injections specifically do so because of weight gain. The other issue with the injection is the possibility of bone thinning with prolonged use. Periods tend to be irregular or absent with these forms of contraception. The absence of periods puts women in a predicament as they worry about pregnancy, although the likelihood is slim given the method's effectiveness. But it's the ideal choice for women who tend to forget to take a daily pill.

Are coils a bit outdated?

No. The older coils, made of copper and without any hormones in, tended to make periods heavier and occasionally more painful. But newer coils – IUCDs or intrauterine contraceptive devices – are incredibly popular and provide excellent contraception, almost as good as sterilisation. They are T-shaped and inserted into the womb via the cervix. The aim is to prevent sperm getting into the uterus by the release of hormones; if they do get there, implantation of the egg and sperm is still unlikely because of the coil. Coils also resolve period problems by making periods at worst a minor spotting event.

Are any other methods available from the doctor?

Yes, patches are available. You apply them weekly for three consecutive weeks, and they work exactly like the combined pill except that the drug goes into the system via the skin. Another clever method is the contraceptive ring, which contains similar hormones. You insert it into the vagina and leave it for three weeks. You go ring-free for one week and then insert one again for the next cycle. Both the patch and the ring are 99 per cent effective.

The morning after pill

This is available over the counter in the UK, Australia and America. It is, however, not the case across Europe so don't get caught out. Remember also that a night of passion can also result in a sexually transmitted infection – and the morning-after pill does not protect against infection. The pill is 95 per effective against pregnancy if taken within twenty-four hours of the encounter, 85 per cent if taken in the second twenty-four hours, but only just above 50/50 if you leave it until seventy-two hours. So make sure you do get it 'the morning after'.

Can I only take it once? No, that's a myth, but it's meant only for emergencies and not long-term contraception. And you should not take it more than once within the same menstrual cycle. Remember your next period may come on time but could be early or late. If it's two weeks late, do a pregnancy test in case the morning-after pill hasn't worked.

Are there any other options if I have left it too late? You can have a coil inserted up to five days after unprotected sex, and this is deemed to be almost 100 per cent effective. It's also an option for anyone who cannot tolerate progesterone, the main ingredient of the morning-after pill.

Tip ▌ *If you vomit within three hours of taking the morning-after pill, it may be ineffective, so take another dose for full protection.*

Other methods

Caps and diaphragms are the way to go if you want to be drug-free. They fit inside the vagina and cover the entrance to the womb. The problem is that they have to be inserted just before sex so some spontaneity is lost. They can also cause irritation and cystitis. The old phrase 'If the cap fits, wear it' holds true here as ill-fitting caps and diaphragms will fail. The overall effectiveness is between 92 and 95 per cent so not as good as other methods.

Tip ▌ *If you pile on 3kg (7lb) or more your cap needs a re-fit, as it may no longer be big enough.*

What's the best post-baby contraception?

If you aren't breastfeeding, you need to think about contraception by the time your baby is twenty-one days old. Exclusive breastfeeding will provide about 98 per cent contraceptive cover, but it's not infallible. If you want to be absolutely sure and continue to feed, choose the mini-pill from day 21. You can also start a patch or implant at this stage if you are not breastfeeding. By four weeks you can consider the coil, and by six weeks you can start injections. Caps and diaphragms can also be used at this stage.

POLYCYSTIC OVARY SYNDROME

This one's far more common than you think, girls, and it often goes undiagnosed. Checklist – acne, excess hair, irregular periods, obesity.

It's due to a fight between the hormones oestrogen and testosterone. The latter isn't just the domain of men; we produce some of this powerful stuff too. The problem in polycystic ovary syndrome – PCOS – is that we have an excess of androgen circulating so, to be blunt, male characteristics emerge and ovulation becomes irregular. The other hormone that comes into play here is insulin, the hormone that goes wrong in diabetes, i.e. it's to do with sugar. In PCOS, the body becomes resistant to insulin and the body begins to produce more insulin to combat this.

How many women suffer, and what do I look out for?

Up to 20 per cent of women of reproductive age suffer from PCOS, but it's likely to be far more as many go undiagnosed. Irregular hair growth, such as inside the thigh, on the nipples or on the chin – generally where you would expect it to sprout in a man – is a feature. Male balding pattern is also seen. The voice can become deep and muscles bulk up. Acne occurs on the face and torso, and the weight tends to be carried around the middle and is difficult to shift.

Menstrual cycles are irregular or absent due to infrequent ovulation. Very often, it's the period problems that cause women to end up at the doctor's questioning their fertility. As periods can be infrequent, this causes alarm in terms of the ability to fall pregnant. To preserve your fertility – as well as your femininity – it's vital that PCOS is tackled head on.

What will the doctor do?

The doctor will very often take a history and might also do some blood tests. These are best done on day 1 to 3 of your cycle. You may also have a scan of your ovaries. PCOS is diagnosed by having any two of the following: polycystic ovaries (usually more than twelve cysts are seen in the ovaries); irregular or a lack of periods; and clinical or biochemical evidence of excess androgen (i.e. blood tests stating that you have too much testosterone, or you're displaying signs, such as facial hair).

What next?

Are you doomed to being hairy and infertile? No you aren't, but it is true to say that the condition cannot be cured. Treatment is based on symptoms and the desire to fall pregnant. Don't ignore it; it won't go away!

▌ Hormonal treatment. The oral contraceptive pill, in particular one with cyproterone in it, works well to cut down the male hormone levels and regulate the menstrual cycle. This pill is ideal if you have acne and body hair and require contraception.

▌ Metformin – a drug used to treat diabetes – restores the balance of insulin and in turn the balance of the male hormones. As a result, periods return in 95 per cent of women.

▌ Eflornithine is a cream, available only on prescription, that gets rid of hair. It does, however, need to be used twice a day, and continuously.

▌ Orlistat may help with weight, and is available over the counter in the UK and Australia.

▌ If you aren't ovulating and are keen to conceive, clomifene (clomiphene) is the drug to get your ovaries working. It acts by stimulating ovulation, i.e. gives your eggs a kickstart. It's normally given under supervision, and you're generally only allowed to have three cycles as it can overstimulate your ovaries.

Surely diet doesn't make a difference as PCOS is due to hormones?

Wrong, diet is of paramount importance here. As many PCOS sufferers are insulin-resistant, high-carbohydrate diets are out as insulin is stimulated mainly by the carbs in your diet. So it's in with the low GI (low glycaemic index) diet. Low GI foods essentially cause a low level of sugar in the bloodstream, which requires lower levels of insulin. It stands to reason that this helps because in PCOS your own insulin is somewhat ineffectual. This will not only pave the way for weight loss, restoration of the menstrual cycle and ovulation, but also help to prevent diabetes in later life.

A low-fat diet is also important as we now know that ladies with PCOS are more likely to develop high cholesterol levels and hardening of the arteries when they are older. So it's important to go high in fibre and low in fat in addition to your carbohydrate counting. Just because the doctor is giving you drugs, don't ditch the diet and exercise plan. It's a vital tool for tackling PCOS.

Will my doctor be aware of this condition?

Don't despair; this is a common problem, and although we aren't sure why it happens, we have been constantly improving our methods of managing since it was first discovered in 1935. Your doctor will have tested and treated female patients for this condition on numerous occasions.

If you are worried, broach the subject with your doctor. In a busy clinic with a backlog, many doctors won't dare broach the subject of body hair or obesity if, for example, you have come in with a bad knee. Physicians often need prompting, so speak up because the bottom line is that your fertility and future health could be at stake. If your PCOS is beyond the scope of your regular doctor, you may be referred to an endocrine specialist, especially if the condition is resistant to treatment or fertility is an issue. Remember though that most PCOS is dealt with in the community.

Tip *Laser hair removal is an option to get rid of the excess facial growth, but it doesn't get rid of the PCOS and its problems, so talk to your doctor.*

CERVICAL CANCER

We're all scared of cervical cancer, yet most of us shun going for a 'smear'. Cervical cancer is on the increase and in the UK is the second most common cancer in women aged between twenty and twenty-nine. Worldwide, one woman dies from it every two minutes. Women in Africa, India and central America are worst affected, predominantly due to their lack of access to screening. We know that 99 per cent of cases are caused by the wart virus, that wart virus transmission isn't blocked by condoms, and that as many as 50 per cent of us have been exposed by our late twenties.

Who is at risk?

Smokers, those who have had a wart virus infection, those with multiple partners from a young age and those with low immunity.

What symptoms might I have?

Sometimes none. But you might have bleeding after sex or between periods – called postcoital and intermenstrual bleeding, respectively – bleeding after the menopause, a smelly vaginal discharge or painful sex.

What does the smear diagnose?

The smear is clever: it diagnoses cells before they become cancerous so doctors can nip them in the bud. Screening with the 'Pap' smear is available free of charge in England and Ireland to those aged over twenty-five, with tests every three years until forty-five and every five years up to sixty. In Australia screening is provided by family doctors with funding through Medicare. They screen every two years, often from age twenty. The American system, although very insurance based, offers free screening to low-income women and advises this to commence at age twenty-one, with tests every three years.

What happens if you've had an abnormal smear?

Some mild changes may be monitored with a repeat test in six months as they usually revert to normal within this time. Don't forget to go back – reminder letters sometimes get lost in the post so mark the date in your diary.

More significant changes are referred for colposcopy. This is a test done under local anaesthetic to survey your cervix with a microscope and stain the cells with acetic acid – vinegar! This shows abnormal cells, which then can be treated by burning or lasering. You may also have a cone biopsy – a cross-sectional slice of the cervix that is viewed under a microscope to establish the extent of the abnormal cells. If they have not penetrated far into your cervix or spread outside it, they can be removed during colposcopy by burning or lasering.

What happens if the cells have gone deep into the cervix?

This usually means surgery – removal of the cervix and womb. Any affected nearby tissues such as the ovaries or lymph glands have to be removed too. And you may need radiotherapy or chemotherapy if the cancer has spread.

Tip *Cervical smears save lives; it's a fact. And the cervical smear test takes about the same time as a TV advertisement break. So are you really too busy for a smear?*

OVARIAN CANCER

Listen carefully ladies as, unlike other cancers, ovarian cancer whispers. It's brutal but it's often caught very late as it creeps up on you. And as five per cent of all cancers in women are ovarian, it ranks as the fifth most common cancer.

Who gets it?

One in ten ovarian cancers are caused by a faulty gene – the BRAC gene, which also increases the risk of breast cancer. If you have breast cancer before the age of forty and a family history of ovarian cancer, you are seventeen times more likely to develop cancer of the ovary.

What else can affect the risks of getting it?

The risk can be increased by HRT, smoking, excess weight, a high-fat diet and never being pregnant. But it will be lowered if you have taken the oral contraceptive pill, have been pregnant or have breastfed.

The symptoms

Listen to your body as this is the only clue. It is only as ovarian cancer grows bigger that you begin to notice things: constant swelling of the abdomen; pain or pressure in the lower abdomen; pain with intercourse; constipation or diarrhoea; back pain; urinary frequency – wanting to go the toilet more often; and occasional and irregular vaginal bleeding. It can grow within the ovary, tubes and womb, and spread to other places, such as the liver, via the blood and lymph. It can also seed tumours into the abdomen, which might show up as a mass in the belly.

How is it diagnosed?

If your history and symptoms are suspicious, you doctor will examine your abdomen and pelvis for any enlargement of the ovaries. You will be sent for an ultrasound scan, and blood tests will be taken to check basic functions as well as the level of CA125, which is an ovarian tumour marker. This gives us more information about activity in the ovary although it doesn't in itself diagnose cancer.

Should I be screened, as with a smear test?

Screening is offered to women with a high-risk history, i.e. those with first-degree relatives with ovarian cancer and those with a personal history of breast cancer at a young age. This involves a CA125 test and ultrasound scan.

Treatment Most women will need surgery to cut out the cancer and anything affected by it. If the tumour is found very late, the surgeon will sometimes only be able to debulk it. Chemotherapy is then used to kill off or shrink down the remaining tumour cells. Ovarian cancer is a destructive disease that is often caught in the late stages. Anyone with symptoms of persistent bloatedness and pelvic pain lasting for more than four weeks should seek advice, and you should consider screening if you have a high-risk family history.

Tip *Beware of new and persistent bloatedness – it may be your ovaries speaking.*

Myth *My smear test was normal so my ovaries must be fine. No – although both come under the heading of gynaecology, they aren't connected.*

WORRIED ABOUT FERTILITY?

Tick tock goes the biological clock. Newspaper headlines tell us we are starting too late, postponing babies to have careers. The truth is that we are twice as fertile in our early twenties as we are in our late thirties and, in obstetric terms, age thirty-five signifies a dramatic decline. There are currently more first-time mothers aged thirty to thirty-four years than twenty-five to twenty-nine in the UK and Ireland, and it's pretty similar for the rest of the developed world. It appears that career women and those with higher educational qualifications are bucking the trend. The Italians wait the longest, with five in every hundred births being to a mum over forty.

Some women spend their early reproductive years being obsessed with contraception and their later years obsessed with conception. Ironically, at a younger age, we're twice as likely to get pregnant as in later years, when we are trying to.

Older mothers

So if you choose to be an older mum, what are the risks? First, you may not fall pregnant. Your chances of pregnancy if you are over forty-five are less than 1 per cent without intervention. The risk of miscarriage is also greater – one in three if you are over forty, but one in ten in your twenties. Chromosomal abnormalities occur more frequently in older mums, with the risks being about one in twenty in a woman over forty-five. Essentially, what this means is that there will be problems with the baby's chromosomes – its genetic make-up – resulting in death, deformity or disability. High blood pressure and diabetes in pregnancy are also more common in older mums, and deliveries are more likely to result in a caesarean section.

What should I do?

Don't panic if your clock is ticking, but do plan ahead. First, gather some information about yourself. Have a blood test to discover if you are immune to rubella (German measles) – you should have had the jab when you were a child, either as part of your MMR vaccination or in school in your teens. It is also important to have a check for Chlamydia and to make sure that your cervical smears are up to date.

Keep a menstrual diary to work out when you are ovulating. Your temperature goes up when you ovulate, and your cervical mucus changes from cloudy to a clear sticky substance like egg white. This signifies your most fertile phase. We often confuse ourselves about ovulation based on our basic knowledge of school biology. We ovulate fourteen days before the onset of bleeding so, for example, if you have a twenty-six day cycle, you ovulate on day twelve, not day fourteen. You can also buy ovulation kits at the pharmacist to check when it's occurring.

What if things are not adding up?

See your doctor for a blood test. You can check your hormone levels at different stages in your cycle, namely follicle stimulating hormone (FSH) and luteinising hormone (LH) at the start of your cycle and progesterone on day twenty-one. Standard bloods tests for thyroid function and basic profiles are also worthwhile. An ultrasound scan will show the condition of your ovaries, and a blood test for anti-müllerian hormone will show your ovarian reserve. This basically gives an indication of how much productivity is left in the ovarian egg factory. It's not always available through your doctor, so you may need to visit a specialist fertility clinic.

What will affect my fertility?

- Stress and emotional strain
- Excess weight loss or weight gain
- Extreme exercising
- Extreme dieting
- A history of Chlamydia or other sexually transmitted infections
- Alcohol consumption outside the safe limits
- Cocaine and marijuana usage
- Thyroid problems
- Long-term medical conditions, such as kidney problems
- Polycystic ovary syndrome
- Endometriosis.

How long will conception take naturally?

Assuming that sexual activity takes place three times a week, eighty-five per cent of couples conceive within the first year of unprotected sex, and 95 per cent within two years. In fact, as many as one in five will fall pregnant after the first month.

How high are my risks of having a Down syndrome child if I postpone pregnancy?

Eighty per cent of babies with Down syndrome are born to mothers under thirty-five. However, at age thirty your risk is one in nine hundred, whereas at forty-five it is one in twenty-five. In addition, you can have as much as a one in five chance of not falling pregnant at all, so rather than concentrate on the negatives, start trying now.

How should I proceed if I'm keen to conceive?

Think seriously about your desire for children – make it the biggest project you have ever undertaken. If you are over thirty-five and want to be a mum but feel the timing isn't right, get checked out so that when the time is right you won't waste it. Meanwhile, look after your mind and body so you are match fit when you finally fall prey to the sperm. It often isn't easy to get pregnant, and pregnancy itself can be a rough ride – and that's even before you begin the eighteen-year stint of raising your babe. So the bottom line is that it is crucial to be in the best physical and mental zone possible. This is one occasion where you cannot 'go with the flow'.

MENOPAUSE

Two words describe the menopause for many women – hot and flush. Menopause designates the passage from virility to sterility. Some women sail through it; others struggle. But like it or not, we all have to face it.

So when will it strike?

The average age is fifty-two, but it can start any time from the mid-forties to the mid-fifties. The levels of the hormones oestrogen and progesterone, which have governed us on a monthly basis for decades, gradually start to crash, and so does our system.

What are the symptoms?

Periods may become light, heavy or irregular, or behave erratically. When they have stopped completely for a full year, that's menopause. The time leading up to this full stop is called the perimenopause, meaning around the menopause. It is during this time that symptoms start.

The hot flush is the classic symptom and can occur about five times a day for as long as two minutes. Heat radiates from the chest to the neck and face, you experience a flush, and you often sweat. The cooling-down period is accompanied by a shiver. Drenching night sweats occur in some women, often needing the sheets to be changed.

Sleep is affected by these flushes, so it may be disturbed or restless. Our intrinsic biological clock seems to shift into a different time zone too. You may have difficulty getting off to sleep, or you may wake at 4am and be unable to go back to sleep. Partners often suffer sleep problems as well as their bed-fellows toss and turn during the night.

The skin becomes less elastic explaining why we become more wrinkled after the menopause. It also loses its moisture and can become dry and flaky. Women sometimes feel that something is crawling on their skin and worry that they have an infestation. The vaginal tissues dry out and, due to this and decreased elasticity, sex can become more painful. The external tissues of the vulva can feel itchy and irritant and look beefy red in appearance. The hair often becomes thinner and drier, and sometimes starts to recede. Facial hair can, however, increase.

The bladder gets more sensitive too, resulting in more frequent attacks of cystitis. Women tend to develop an expert knowledge of the locations of public toilets due to the decrease in bladder capacity, and they can suffer leakage when coughing or laughing.

Generalised aches and pains occur in the joints and muscles The zest for life is sometimes zapped and replaced with lethargy and tiredness. Mood can be affected, ranging from depression to anxiety and panic attacks. Women who suffer from premenstrual syndrome are more likely to become depressed around the menopause. And libido seems to lessen, which, compounded with other features, can affect relationships.

Menopause sounds like pure misery. What should I do?

First, find out if it is menopause. Other problems – diabetes, thyroid dysfunction, anaemia, depression – may be implicated. A blood test can be done if the diagnosis is in doubt. An elevated blood level of the hormone FSH is diagnostic of menopause, but not every woman needs a blood test as menopause is often straightforward to diagnose from the symptoms. Do remember, however, that irregular bleeding can be due to other causes, like polyps, fibroids or problems with the womb's lining, so don't pin everything on the menopause. A new onset of night sweats can be a sinister sign, indicating tuberculosis, malaria or even lymphoma. The golden rule is to go and talk to a doctor you like as significant medical problems may be missed behind the mask of menopause. Every woman is different.

Self-help

We like a bit of self-help. Exercise is of paramount importance. It boosts energy and libido. Weightbearing exercise such as walking is also brilliant for maintaining bone density and preventing osteoporosis. Exercise helps with weight gain too – we need to be particularly conscious of the circumference around the belly button. Ladies who exceed more than 80cm (31.5in) here put themselves at increased risk of developing diabetes. The cholesterol level also shoots up during menopause so watch the fats. Remember to eat your five portions of fruit and vegetables a day to get your antioxidants, and make sure there is enough calcium in your diet for your bones, and enough iron to give you energy. Postmenopausal ladies are often deficient in these nutrients.

Male patients have described their wives to me as miserable menopausal mares. You don't have to be one, and for many women menopause is a liberating journey that starts a new phase of life. Our grandmothers put up and shut up, but we don't have to – empower yourself to seek help. Talk to your doctor about all of the aspects of your menopause and together work out a management plan. Interestingly, men have their own menopause, called andropause, but they just don't care to admit it.

HRT – DOES IT HELP?

HRT, standing for hormone replacement therapy and unfortunately not for hardcore retail therapy, can make you feel like some kind of oestrogen addict. But hormone replacement therapy really does what it says on the tin – replaces the dwindling stores of oestrogen. The menopause is cold turkey time in terms of hormonal withdrawal, and HRT serves to steer you through it by topping up your hormone levels. The general consensus of opinion is that if it is used for five years or less, its benefits outweigh its risks in suitable patients.

That seems sensible, so why all the hulabaloo?

HRT isn't risk-free. Studies have proven that there is a link between taking HRT and breast cancer. There are two factors to take note of here. Women who take HRT for ten years have a greater risk of this, as do women who take combined HRT, i.e. one that replaces the two hormones oestrogen and progesterone. So how do the numbers add up? Well, for every thousand women taking only oestrogen for five years, there will be two extra cases of breast cancer. If they take it for ten years, there will be six extra cases of breast cancer. Taking combined HRT for five years results in six extra cases of breast cancer, and for ten years, twenty-four extra cases.

Would we knowingly take something that can cause cancer? No. However, it is important to be aware that the symptoms of menopause can be very severe and debilitating, and the benefits to a patient sometimes outweigh the small but not insignificant risks.

Quick stats

The risk of ovarian cancer is one in a hundred if you take any type of HRT for ten years. The risk of stroke is one in a thousand if HRT is taken for five years, and double that if it is taken for ten. Blood clots will occur in two in one thousand women taking oestrogen-only HRT for five years, and in seven in one thousand women taking combined treatments. The bottom line is to consider the stats before you act and don't stay on HRT for longer than five years if possible.

Who can't have HRT?

Any woman with a history of breast cancer, ovarian cancer or cancer of the womb, with heart disease or high blood pressure, with a history of blood clots, with liver disease or with a history of stroke.

Read all the pros and cons, and fancy a go at HRT?

Book a prearranged appointment to see your doctor, and take the time to discuss your options. You don't have to come away from the consultation with a prescription – you can have a think and decide. There are numerous options available, ranging from tablets and cream gels to patches, implants and pessaries.

Treatments for those still having periods or who have only just stopped

You need to take oestrogen every day and progesterone for fourteen days every month to allow an artificial monthly bleed. You can also use a three-monthly preparation whereby you bleed every quarter. You must have this artificial period to allow the lining of the womb to break down until it is fully established that you are menopausal, i.e. you have had no periods for one full year. If you have had a hysterectomy, you will only need to take oestrogen.

Bleed-free HRT is given to women who have not had a period for a year or who are fifty-four or over. This daily combination of oestrogen and progesterone does not involve a withdrawal bleed so is far more convenient. Tibolone, available in some countries, is a synthetic hormone that mimics the effect of oestrogen, progesterone and testosterone. It works well in terms of controlling menopausal symptoms, and the additional testosterone kick can give women a bit of a libido boost.

If your main bother is vaginal dryness, painful sex and bladder problems, try topical HRT. You insert this yourself and it delivers hormone locally into the vaginal tissue, so there are no general side-effects and no bleeding.

Follow-up

It goes without saying that you can't reach for HRT and grow old gracefully without check-ups. You will need to continue breast screening, smear tests, bone scans for osteoporosis and regular blood pressure and follow-up checks at the doctors every six months. You are unlikely to be on HRT for more than five years, and many women stop renewing their prescription after two years as by this stage most of the symptoms will have disappeared. Take care when coming off HRT though: don't go cold turkey – it's best to wean yourself off it to avoid any withdrawal effects.

Tip ▌ *Having a mammogram may be like slamming your breast in the garage door, but a mammogram may save your life, particularly if you are menopausal and on HRT. Don't decline the invitation to attend.*

PROLAPSE

The word prolapse literally means to fall out of place, and that's exactly what happens, ladies, when our pelvic floors let us down. It is estimated that one in eight of us succumb to gravity and suffer from a prolapse. This results in structures such as the uterus, vagina, bowel and bladder falling out of their normal positions. Imagine your pelvic floor like a paper shopping bag. If part of it becomes weak, bits of your shopping may poke out or fall out. But rather than saying things are falling out or dropping down, doctors tend to medicalise it by using the word descent.

Is it a design fault or does something actually cause prolapse?

Anything that weakens the pelvic scaffolding can cause prolapse – one of the chief causes is weakening and stretching of the muscles and ligaments during pregnancy and delivery. As we age, our hormone levels dip, and in a similar way to our skin losing its structure, so does our pelvic floor, especially during the menopause. Some people are genetically more predisposed to it. In addition, anything that puts extra pressure on the abdomen can contribute, so that means excess weight or chronic coughing in heavy smokers.

Could my womb literally fall out? What would happen?

It's actually more a question of dropping down rather than falling out. Divide your pelvis mentally into three – front, middle and back. Your symptoms depend on where the weakness is. If the front section of muscle becomes weak, it's the bladder and water pipe that are affected. They can protrude into the vagina and give you symptoms with your waterworks. If the middle section is up to mischief, it is possible that the womb, the walls of the vagina or a small portion of bowel may protrude. And if the back third of the pelvic floor is affected, it's all about your back passage, with a portion of the rectum falling forward into the vagina.

What's the most likely to occur?

Prolapse of the bladder is the most common form, followed by prolapse of the womb, followed by the back passage. If the bladder is affected, the symptoms are usually wetting when you cough or sneeze or can't get to the toilet quickly enough. You may also feel a need to pass urine frequently and sense that you haven't emptied your bladder properly. This leaves you with a mixed picture of incontinence and an overactive bladder.

Where the bowel or rectum (back passage) is involved, it often results in constipation, an urgent call to stool or a feeling that you haven't 'emptied' properly. Other problems that crop up are pain or discomfort with sex, a feeling of pressure or a sensation that something is dropping down. Passing 'wind' out the front end of your pelvis can also be a symptom.

How does the doctor diagnose this?

You will need to talk your doctor through your symptoms and how they are affecting your day-to-day life. Your doctor will then examine you, not like they would for a smear but with you rolled over onto your left side. They may ask you to strain as if you are passing a motion, and this will highlight any prolapse.

Can it be treated?

Treatment depends on you and how it is affecting your life. A prolapse isn't usually life-threatening, but it can definitely be life-impacting. If your bowels call too often, you're struggling with your sex life or you're never out without an incontinence pad, a visit to a gynaecologist might be on the cards.

Surgical options depend on the site of the prolapse and, contrary to many women's worries, do not always involve a hysterectomy. The issue with surgery is that the poor pelvic floor that gave you the prolapse in the first place is still present, and you can end up with a further prolapse elsewhere. About one in four women find they need a further operation.

Are there any other options?

Tackle excess weight, smoking and constipation as they may be making your prolapse worse, and if you come to need an operation, these issues will need to be dealt with anyway. Pelvic floor exercises may help you. It is always best to be taught these by a trained physiotherapist as we often squeeze the wrong muscles and get no benefit.

Ring pessaries These are plastic or silicone devices a bit like a child's bangle. They come in all shapes and sizes and are tucked up into the vagina, where they provide support to the structures. Your family doctor can usually fit these, and they need to be changed every three to six months. This might suit you better than surgery or can be used as a stop-gap before an operation. If they are going to fall out, this usually happens when you get off the doctor's couch. So as a general rule, if it's in, you don't need to worry as it's likely to stay in.

If I haven't got a prolapse, how can I prevent getting one?

Pelvic floor exercises are vital not only after childbirth, but also during pregnancy. Weight is another factor – pile on the pounds and prolapse is more likely. And avoid anything that puts too much pressure on, such as lifting heavy weights or becoming chronically constipated.

So should everybody be doing a pelvic floor workout?

Yes, in an effort to prevent and control urinary symptoms and prepare the pelvis for childbirth, and then restore it after childbirth. Like all exercise, there is no quick fix. Kegel exercises were developed by an American obstetrician named Arnold Kegel; the secret of their success is in knowing what to squeeze!

The biggest mistake women make is in thinking they know what muscles to tighten, so here's how you locate your 'pelvics'. Put simply, you squeeze your pelvic floor muscle when you stop your urinary flow midstream or if you're trying to inhibit the passage of gas. You can choose to do the exercises lying, sitting or even standing at the kitchen sink. Contract the muscles and hold for three seconds, then relax for three seconds and, as you would do in the gym, try ten repetitions. Gradually build up to four seconds, the aim being to squeeze for a full ten seconds, doing ten repetitions three times a day. As with all exercise, it may take eight to twelve weeks before you tone up.

Need an instructor?

Good urogynaecological physiotherapists are worth their weight in gold. They can literally train your pelvic muscles. Another helping hand comes in the form of a pelvic toner. There are many devices that can be inserted which stimulate your pelvic floor muscles to tighten –weights, cones, sprung devices and muscular stimulators. Some look like hair straighteners – but don't be put off by their appearance. Give them a go and you will be pleasantly surprised.

What if I think I might have a prolapse?

See your doctor, discuss your symptoms and have an examination. The diagnosis does not require any tests as it is done with the naked eye. As this condition is so common, your doctor will have seen it hundreds of times before. Even if you don't think you have a prolapse, you haven't had a baby or you see menopause as something that is decades away, start doing pelvic floor exercises and beat the almost inevitable descent of later life.

Tips
- *Pelvic floor exercises will not only help prevent prolapse, but also improve your sex life.*
- *Pelvic floor exercises help everyone, even your man! Do them together as it will help his erectile function and bladder control too.*

Breasts

3

This chapter deals with all matters mammary – important reading for every woman.

BREAST EXAMINATION

Rather than getting bogged down with this, the key here is to know what's normal for *you*. With our lifetime risk of getting breast cancer lying at one in nine, there's a high probability that you are at some point going to find a lump, be it benign or malignant.

Get checking

The worst possible time to check your breasts is just before or during your period because your breasts are sore and swollen. Ideally, do it one week after your period. But remember that you are probably doing a mini-check every day in the bath and the shower when you wash, and this is often when ladies notice lumps.

HOW TO EXAMINE YOUR BREASTS

Lie down on your back with one hand behind your head. Use your free hand to examine your opposite breast, following the instructions overleaf.

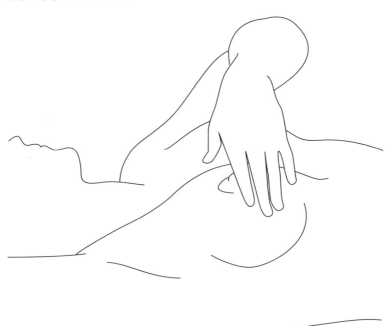

Look Take a good look in front of the mirror. You are looking for asymmetry, puckered skin, eczematous changes or redness. Are the nipples turning inwards? Is there swelling or an irregular shape?

Feel Lie down on your back with one hand behind your head. Use your free hand to examine your opposite breast. Your fingers are the sensors, so start to feel with a flat hand and the second, third and fourth fingers. These serve as your rudder to guide you around the breast. I tend to start at the outside and work inwards in a circular motion. Apply gentle pressure initially and then go deep.

Examinations

If you find anything at all, see your doctor. It is far better to be reassured than to worry unnecessarily. Mammograms are generally done in the over fifties. However, they are not foolproof and may miss 10 per cent of cancers. The breast tissue in young women is often dense, so if you're under forty, you will be advised to have an ultrasound scan or an MRI (magnetic resonance imaging) scan. The chief tool in the detection of all lumps is clinical examination as a skilled practitioner can tell the difference between a safe lump and a sinister one.

THERE'S A LUMP IN MY BREAST

What could it be?

First, most breast lumps aren't cancers. Eight out of every ten lumps that end up at the doctors are benign, but that's NO EXCUSE for not getting checked out. The breast has a network of glands, ducts, nerves, fat cells and blood vessels, all of which can cause mischief.

First up, the fibroadenoma

This one always worries women as it tends to feel quite firm. It occurs most often in your twenties and feels like a smooth lump under the skin. You find it and then it seems to move under your finger or disappear – that's why we refer to it as a 'breast mouse'.

It can become quite large, but the average fibroadenoma is normally no bigger than your thumbnail. The doctor is likely to send you for a mammogram or ultrasound to confirm the diagnosis.

If the lump isn't bothering you, you don't usually need to do anything about it. Fibroadenomas tend to stop growing after two to three years and in about 10 per cent of cases just disappear. If the lump is painful, the diagnosis is in doubt or you are over forty, you can have a minor operation to remove it. Fibroadenomas can, however, reoccur after surgery.

Next, fibrocystic disease

This is very common and shouldn't really be called a 'disease' as 50 per cent of women in their thirties and forties suffer from it at some point. If the trio of adjectives lumpy, heavy and painful sum up your breasts, this could be your problem.

During the monthly cycle, the breast reacts as if it is preparing for pregnancy, just like the womb. And when you don't fall pregnant, a similar process of breaking things down also occurs in the breast. So individuals with fibrocystic breast disease often experience symptoms in the second half of their cycle. The difficulty with this condition is that, because it gives rise to generally lumpy breasts, self-examination can be a struggle. Looking for a lump is like looking for a rock in a sea of gravel. So know what's normal for you and have a check-up every six months with your doctor.

Breast cysts

Breast cysts can appear as painful lumps that can become tender and grow as big as an orange. On the other hand, some women do not notice any pain or bumpiness until a lump is picked up on examination. Cysts are caused by hormone fluctuations during the menstrual cycle and can also be caused by hormone replacement therapy (HRT).

The lump will feel jelly-like, and you may be able to poke your finger into its centre. A cyst is usually confirmed by either ultrasound testing in young women or a mammogram in over thirty-fives. The specialist is likely to drain the fluid off if a diagnosis is needed or the cyst is uncomfortable.

Fat necrosis

The breast contains lots of fat cells, which is one reason our breasts grow bigger when we gain weight. Any trauma to the breast can damage a portion of this fatty tissue. You may not recall any injury but may find a firm, round lump that can cause redness on the breast surface. The doctor will send you to have the diagnosis confirmed by a specialist. The good news is that it tends to disappear of its own accord.

Lipoma

This feels like a round, firm lump and can occur any where in the breast. You will often find lipomas elsewhere, for example the abdominal wall. They are essentially just blobs of fat in the breast that are encapsulated (surrounded by a covering) – think chocolate-coated raisins. Lipomas can be difficult to diagnose so often warrant a scan. As lipomas are benign, they do not need to be removed unless the diagnosis is in doubt or they become very large or painful.

MY BREASTS ACHE

Why does it happen?

We are conditioned to think that if something hurts, something sinister is going on, but breast pain – mastalgia – isn't usually a symptom of breast cancer. Seventy per cent of us suffer from pain at some point but, like many medical conundrums, there are no concrete answers to why it happens.

Our amazing breasts

Our breasts are in a constant state of flux throughout our menstrual cycle. They contain fat, support fibres and lots of glands. Each month these glands prepare to make milk as every cycle has the possibility of pregnancy. The breasts are stimulated by two hormones, oestrogen and progesterone, during the second half of your cycle, after you have ovulated. These can make the breasts swell and the glands engorge, so your breasts feel tender. But this doesn't mean anything is wrong – some women just have more sensitive breast tissue.

Men don't get this pain as they aren't governed by fluctuating monthly hormones. This makes it difficult for them to fathom that their objects of desire can be the cause of excruciating discomfort for two weeks every month!

Hormones

We tend to call pain that occurs with the menstrual cycle cyclical breast pain. It's most common in young women between thirty and fifty. One or both sides can be affected, and it tends to hurt most in the upper outer part of the breast and the inner aspect of the arm. It's worst three to five days before your period and can be so severe it's impossible to wear tight clothing; it may even be necessary to wear a bigger bra.

Treatment Keep a symptom diary in order to work out how the pain affects you. Simple painkillers like ibuprofen and paracetamol can help. The oral contraceptive pill may be an option if contraception is needed as it can decrease cyclical pain and swelling. There is evidence that decreasing caffeine, animal fat and salt intake may help too. Some women find a diet high in soy, vitamin B6 and vitamin E to be beneficial; others swear by magnesium supplements. Water tablets (diuretics) and gamolenic acid or evening primrose oil used to be favourite treatments, but there is not much evidence to support them. The evidence on what works in terms of supplements and diet is fairly vague, but if it's safe and seems to help, stick with it.

Serious drugs can be considered too – these include medicines that block hormones, like tamoxifen (used in breast cancer), danazol (used in the treatment of endometriosis) and bromocriptine (used to stop milk production after childbirth). But these are a last resort as they have significant side-effects.

How long does breast pain go on for?

It can disappear after three to six months, but in over half of these cases it can come back within a couple of years.

What if it isn't related to my cycle?

We cleverly call this non-cyclical breast pain, and it tends to strike women in their forties. The cause may not be clear, but pain may come from the breast, chest wall or adjoining nerves and muscles. It's generally one-sided. Breast cancer needs to be ruled out in the case of persistent pain: about one in twenty women with breast cancer will report pain as a symptom.

Tips
▌ *Have a specific well-fitting 'breastache bra' to wear during the sore time of your cycle.*

▌ *Ditch the underwire in favour of the more supportive sports number. You can wear it during sleep too.*

▌ *Remember that although HRT and the pill may help breast pain, they can also cause it. And breast pain in your forties may be the first sign that you are approaching menopause.*

Breast pain presents two main problems: the inconvenience of the pain itself and the underlying worry of something sinister. As with all matters mammary, see your doctor. Bring a symptom diary to help gauge how bad it is, and try to go when it you can be examined without too much pain. If your symptoms persist, don't put up with it – go back. It never hurts to be reassured a second time.

DISCHARGE FROM THE NIPPLE

The vast majority of women who experience discharge from the nipple do not have cancer. But that doesn't let you off the hook – if the nipple is discharging, book a doctor's appointment.

What are worrying signs?

▌ Discharge from one nipple only

▌ Blood-stained discharge

▌ Persistent discharge

▌ You are over forty and have a lump in your breast.

What's going on?

Both sides leaking? Milky discharge from both breasts can occur from stimulation, tight clothing or even exercise. Up to two years post pregnancy, women will often have a milky discharge on hearing a baby cry or on touching the nipple area – that's normal. Medicines that you are taking can sometimes cause the problem too, for example cimetidine, which is an ulcer medicine, some antidepressants, the oral contraceptive pill and some over-the-counter antinausea medications.

A prolactinoma is a growth in the pituitary gland in your brain that causes an excess of the hormone prolactin (literally meaning 'pro lactation'). This hormone is normally produced after childbirth. A milky discharge from both nipples can be a sign that you have a prolactinoma; it may also be accompanied by headache, visual symptoms and irregular or absent periods. We call this milky discharge galactorrhoea when it's unrelated to breastfeeding. Bloody discharge can occur from both breasts during pregnancy and breastfeeding

One side leaking? It is possible that you have a papilloma. Don't panic – these are benign little growths in the milk duct system and can cause a milky discharge from one breast. The milk ducts can also become inflamed, which results in discharge. One-sided nipple discharge even in the absence of a lump can, however, be a sign of breast cancer, particularly in those over forty.

What happens next?

Doctors often send the fluid that is expressed from the nipple for an analysis of the cells and to check it for blood or infection. They are likely to refer you for a mammogram or an ultrasound scan of the breast if you are over forty or have a blood-stained discharge. If you can elicit the discharge by stimulating the nipples and it's milky, it is far less likely to be sinister. In this instance, the doctor will often refer you for blood tests to check for hormone imbalance, in particular the level of the hormone prolactin that I mentioned above.

If you have a growth or an inflammation in the milk duct system, it may be necessary to have a minor surgical procedure to cut the duct out. This is a simple procedure and does not affect nursing a baby or nipple sensation afterwards.

What if I am found to be making too much prolactin?

About one in ten thousand people have a prolactinoma – the benign tumour that produces too much of this prolactin stuff. This leads to discharging nipples, visual symptoms and headache. If it is a small growth, it's often left alone, but if the symptoms are bothersome or you're trying to fall pregnant, medication can be used. If the prolactinoma is very large, you may need to have an operation. The first two solutions are, however, the norm.

The bottom line

Nipple discharge should not be ignored – although it is unlikely, there is an outside possibility that it could be a sign of breast cancer. So get it checked.

BREAST CANCER

Think of nine of your closest female friends. One of them is likely to get breast cancer. Statistically, the risk is one in nine in a woman's lifetime, and yes, that's shockingly high.

What increases our risk?

Both men and women have breast tissue, yet breast cancer in men accounts for only 1 per cent of breast tumours. So being female is top of the list.

Hormones also play a role. Hormone replacement therapy (HRT) increases the risks too. In addition, the risk is increased with age, which is why we see most cases in the over fifties. Oral contraceptive pill users have a slightly increased risk too, but this disappears ten years after stopping the pill. However, it's also important to remember that using the pill reduces the risk of ovarian cancer.

Lifestyle issues are a factor in breast cancer. Obesity and excess alcohol consumption both increase your risk. Where you chose to live has an impact too – there are more breast cancer cases in Scandinavia, for example, than in the UK. Women who do not have children or bear their first child after thirty have an increased risk of breast cancer, as do those with an early onset of menstruation and a late menopause.

The family tree features here as well, with a higher incidence in those with a first-degree relative with breast or ovarian cancer, particularly if this occurred before the age of 50. If you yourself have had ovarian cancer, your risk of breast cancer shoots up to seventeen times the average.

What should I be on the look out for?

Be breast aware. Any change, no matter how small, needs checking.

The danger signs are:

- If the shape of your breast changes
- If the nipple turns inward, discharges or becomes irritated
- If the skin puckers
- If your armpit feels sore
- If you feel any change in the shape or consistency of your breast.

Know what's normal for you and remember that any deviation from this warrants a visit to the doctor. It is the doctor's job, and not yours, to decide what's safe and what isn't.

Found a lump or noticed a change?

The majority of breast lumps are not cancerous, but they all warrant a doctor's review. A cancerous lump generally feels hard and irregular and is likely to be immobile.

What happens next?

If your doctor finds something, you will be referred to a breast clinic and usually seen and assessed within two weeks. This clinic will often be what is called a one-stop-shop. This means that you get seen by a specialist, who will then advise on the type of scan you need.

- This may be a mammogram, which is the most commonly used screening test.
- Ultrasound scans are used to assess and locate fluid-filled lumps.
- MRI scanning – magnetic resonance imaging, to give it its full name – is sometimes used in young women.

Based on the images obtained, you may require a biopsy, which is where an instrument like an apple corer is inserted into the breast to remove a sample of tissue. Fluid might also be drawn off by means of inserting a needle. These procedures are done under local anaesthetic, and larger samples can be taken under general anaesthetic if they are needed. These samples are then sent to the lab for analysis. It is on the basis of this analysis that the diagnosis is made and treatment prescribed.

What kind of treatment is done?

First, the tumour is 'graded' to describe how abnormal it looks. It is defined as low, intermediate or high grade. High-grade cells will grow more quickly and may return after treatment. The tumour is also 'staged' to work out how far it has grown or spread, for example outside the breast.

Most of the time, the first stage of treatment is surgery, either to remove the cancer and the surrounding healthy area, or to remove the whole breast. If the lump alone is removed, radiotherapy is used to prevent problems in the rest of the breast. If you have a high-grade cancer, you may be advised to have chemotherapy after surgery to prevent recurrence. Each woman is different depending on the type of cancer, her age and where the cancer is situated, so that is what dictates the treatment.

Is there anything else?

You will be tested to see whether you have oestrogen receptors on the cancer cells. Many breast cancers grow in response to oestrogen, and have these receptors on their surface that attract oestrogen like a magnet; this in turn stimulates the cancer to grow. Hormone therapy that interferes with this, such as tamoxifen, can be used before surgery to shrink the tumour or afterwards to prevent its recurrence in suitable patients.

Follow-up

You will be followed up on a regular basis for at least five years, and if you're clear at this stage, you can generally speaking consider yourself free of disease. It is vital, however, to continue to have checks as cancers can come back or crop up in the other breast.

BREAST REDUCTION

Breasts come in all shapes and sizes; not even our own two are the same! We live in a consumer society where anyone can 'buy new boobs', and we are bombarded with the media perception that bigger is better. Breast augmentation is often sought by those who want more fulfillment or whose breasts have shrunk after weight loss or childbirth. Ironically, many women need to do the opposite. The big breasts bestowed upon you in pregnancy may never go down, or you may be genetically predisposed to a bigger chest – thanks, Gran.

When bigger isn't always better

A big cup size and the extra weight can bring physical problems of back, neck and shoulder pain. Poor posture, breathing difficulties, and soreness under the breast and in the region of bra straps can also be a problem. And there can be psychological difficulties such as feeling self-conscious or constantly being identified in terms of your assets. Sporting activities are restricted and clothing options limited. Primarily, the problem is a disproportionate relationship between the physical weight of the breasts and the size of the body frame – carrying around several extra kilograms can be downright tiring.

What happens in breast reduction?

If you are suitable, the procedure – mammoplasty – will be carried out under general anaesthetic and may take three to four hours. The surgeon removes skin, breast and fat tissue to resize and reshape the breast. An anchor-shaped cut is made starting at the nipple and extending downwards and then horizontally. The nipple is generally left in place, but if there is lots of excess tissue, the nipple will be removed and replaced higher using a skin graft. A vertical scar reduction involves a cut around the nipple and then just vertically, meaning there is no scarring underneath the breast.

Problems

Most surgery will result in minor differences in scar size and breast shape. Wound infection and bleeding can be a problem too. Loss of nipple sensation and the ability to breastfeed generally occur only if the nipple is actually removed and replaced – usually only if the breasts are exceptionally large. Temporary loss of nipple and skin sensation may occur with standard procedures but are usually restored by twelve weeks.

You are likely to be in hospital for one or two nights and should be back at work in up to a fortnight. You will have quite a bit of bruising, which will gradually fade after a few weeks. The first image of the breasts after the operation is often cosmetically better than that a few days later when the swelling starts to go down and the bruising appears. The final result may take may months to become apparent.

Cosmetic surgery tourism

Every woman wants a bargain, but every woman also deserves the best. No procedure is risk-free, but at least if you stay on home turf you will have someone on hand in case of any complications. Air travel and major surgery increase the risk of potentially fatal blood clots, especially if you smoke, take hormones or are over forty; and the longer you are immobile through surgery or air travel, the greater your risk.

So have your surgery carried out by a surgeon registered with the General Medical Council plastic surgery register and the British Association of Plastic, Reconstructive and Aesthetic Surgeons, the Michelin stars in terms of plastic surgeons. And don't randomly pick a specialist out of the phone book – you wouldn't have your highlights done by a random stranger, so don't plump for a surgical specialist on a whim. Flashy adverts don't always equate with the best outcome. Do your research and inform your doctor of your intentions. They can advise you on 'the good, the bad and the ugly' of cosmetic surgery.

Tips   *Don your shock-absorbent sports bra for six weeks after the operation and avoid vigorous physical activity. This prevents discomfort and allows the 'new' breasts to convalesce.*

     If you intend breastfeeding, postpone the operation as you may not be able to breastfeed, or you may be left with large post-pregnancy breasts and be back where you started.

Circulation

4

This is what gets our blood pumping, and keeps us all from keeling over. Check up on the common cardiovascular ailments and tips for a healthy heart.

BLOOD PRESSURE

We have all heard of blood pressure, but do any of us really know what it's about? Well, it's the pressure that the circulating blood exerts on the walls of blood vessels and is measured in millimetres of mercury. Clear as mud, isn't it?

Imagine water running through a hose pipe – the greater the water pressure exerted by turning the tap, the faster the water flows and the more pressure it puts on the hose. The lower the pressure, the slower the flow. As a result, very high pressures may damage the hose, and equally, high blood pressure damages our blood vessels.

What causes high blood pressure?

Doctors refer to high blood pressure as hypertension, but they generally use the abbreviation BP. In 95 per cent of cases, we call this raised blood pressure essential hypertension because we don't truly know why it happens. Rather surprisingly, we can find a reason in only about 5 per cent of cases, for example kidney disease, problems with the adrenal glands, pregnancy and the oral contraceptive pill.

WHAT IS THE AVERAGE BLOOD PRESSURE RANGE FOR YOUR AGE?

Age range	Average blood pressure	Minimum blood pressure	Maximum blood pressure
20–24	120 / 79	108 / 75	132 / 83
25–29	121 / 80	109 / 76	133 / 84
30–34	122 / 81	110 / 77	134 / 85
35–39	123 / 82	111 / 78	135 / 86
40–44	125 / 83	112 / 79	137 / 87
45–49	127 / 84	115 / 80	139 / 88
50–54	129 / 85	116 / 81	142 / 89
55–59	131 / 86	118 / 82	144 / 90
60–64	134 / 87	121 / 83	147 / 91

What makes me more likely to suffer from this?

- If you have a family history of high blood pressure
- If you smoke
- If you are of African-American origin
- If you are pregnant or on the pill
- If you are overweight or obese
- If you don't exercise
- If you consume too much alcohol
- If you eat a high-salt diet
- If you abuse cocaine or amphetamines.

But if I have high blood pressure, I can just see my doctor and get it fixed, right?

Yes, but unfortunately the most dangerous aspect of high blood pressure is that you may not have any symptoms. Symptoms can include headache, dizziness, tiredness and nosebleeds, but often you are symptom-free – that's why we call it the silent killer.

How is it checked?

It's easy to check blood pressure by means of a special piece of kit called a sphygmomanometer. This is a cuff that inflates on your arm and measures the pressure in a blood vessel. The doctor notes two readings: the first represents the systolic blood pressure, and the second the diastolic blood pressure. The systolic pressure is the pressure of the blood when the heart contracts to push the blood round the body. The diastolic pressure is the pressure of the blood when the heart is resting. We then document these numbers as the systolic reading over the diastolic reading, so that your doctor might, for example, say 120 over 80mmHg.

It's a numbers game

The average blood pressure is 120 over 80. We call your blood pressure high if it reads 140 over 90 or greater. But this would never be diagnosed based on one reading alone, so your doctor may ask you to return at varying intervals over a few weeks to check it.

What's white coat syndrome?

Some women (and men too) get anxious when they visit the doctor, and this puts their blood pressure up. It then tends to be a vicious circle as worrying about your blood pressure being high then makes it high. If you're going for a check, get there on time and chill out in the waiting room for ten minutes before your appointment. If you need to go to the toilet, go, as wanting to spend a penny may increase your BP. Don't have your car on a meter or a chicken in the oven, otherwise you will feel stressed. You may think that relaxing with a cigarette or a coffee will give you a better score, but it won't – caffeine and nicotine both increase blood pressure.

Is it me or the doctor?

A handsome male doctor can undoubtedly affect your blood pressure! However, if the diagnosis is in doubt after several attempts, you will be advised to have twenty-four-hour blood pressure monitoring over the course of a day, even when you are asleep. The monitor is like a personal stereo recording device with a blood pressure cuff. You can now also buy effective digital home monitors at pharmacies, so you can take your blood pressure at your leisure, such as watching television.

The next step

It's not pills straight away for high blood pressure, so don't panic. If your BP is only borderline, it is safe to try other measures initially. First, look at your diet. Limit your salt intake to under 6g a day – that's a teaspoonful. Beware because even though you might not add salt, soups, ready meals and crisps are full of it, so always read the label. Opt too for low-fat and high-fibre foods.

If you are overweight, it's imperative to address this. Try to exercise for thirty minutes a day at least five times a week. But not just strolling round the shops – it should involve increasing your heart rate and getting out of puff. Eliminate or limit your alcohol consumption by drinking less than fourteen units a week and ensuring you have alcohol-free days. It goes without saying that you should stop smoking.

Tests If it is established that you have high blood pressure, you will be advised to have blood tests to check for cholesterol level, diabetes and kidney function. You are also likely to be asked to have a urine test and possibly a heart tracing (called an ECG or EKG). Depending on the results, you may be referred to a cardiologist, but most blood pressure problems can be managed by your family doctor.

Treatment   Numerous medical treatments are available. Generally, you will be advised treatment if your blood pressure is consistently 160 over 100 or more, aiming to get it under control and prevent complications. Reducing your diastolic blood pressure can reduce your chances of having a stroke by 34 per cent. For many people, treatment is lifelong, but if your medicine has kept your blood pressure low for several years, there may be an option to come off it. But don't just 'decide' to come off your medication – discuss it with your doctor. There are many different combinations of treatment, and although they may not make you feel any different on the outside, rest assured that they are working hard on the inside.

Why it needs to be treated

High blood pressure is unlikely to affect you in your daily life right now, but if uncontrolled it could affect you in the future. Failure to control your blood pressure may result in complications including strokes, heart attacks, kidney failure and blindness.

Low blood pressure

This is common in ladies and is not serious like high blood pressure. It can make you feel faint or dizzy if you jump out of bed suddenly or get out of a warm bath. Make sure you keep well hydrated and avoid sudden changes in posture. Standing for long periods in a warm room at a drinks party may prove problematic as the combination of standing, heat, alcohol and low blood pressure makes you more likely to faint.

Tips   *If your blood pressure pills are giving you side-effects, speak up – don't just stop taking them.*
One in three adults in the Western world has high blood pressure at some point. Have a check every three to five years if you are under fifty and every year if you are over fifty.

Myth   *Doctors only check your blood pressure when you are on the pill because they get paid for it. Wrong – we do it because blood pressure is one of the serious side-effects of the pill that can occur at any stage while you are taking it.*

CHOLESTEROL

LEVELS OF CHOLESTEROL

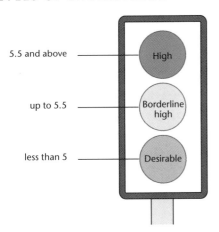

5.5 and above —— High

up to 5.5 —— Borderline high

less than 5 —— Desirable

Cholesterol is a fatty substance found in the bloodstream and in every cell in the body. Although it's vital for survival as it plays a role in important bodily functions, too much of it is a bad thing.

Why is it such a problem?

High levels of cholesterol cause fat to be deposited in our blood vessels, hindering blood flow. This affects important organs such as the brain and heart, and can result in stroke and heart attacks. Bits of fat can also break free and plug a blood vessel downstream, with the same results.

What affects the fat balance?

Smoking, obesity, a poor diet – one high in animal fat and artificial fats called trans fats – lack of exercise, high blood pressure, diabetes and a family history of high cholesterol can all help to tip the fat balance from good to bad.

Know your score

Two out of every three adults have a higher than recommended cholesterol. Do you know yours? It should be 5mmol/l or under. In addition, your cholesterol should be predominantly of the HDL (high-density lipoprotein) variety because, although cholesterol is deemed bad, some of it does good work, and this is the HDL cholesterol. Cholesterol that is damaging to the heart is called LDL (low-density lipoprotein) cholesterol; your level of this should be less than 3. Your goal is a cholesterol level within the normal range with a low LDL and a high HDL.

Fat-busting tips

Watch the fat. Make sure you get no more than 10 per cent of your calories from saturated fat. Simple measures like using olive oil instead of vegetable oil can help. Think about trans fats, which lie hidden in margarine and snacks – these increase your LDL and lower your HDL, so it's double trouble. The clue is on the label – if the product contains a partially hydrogenated oil, that's a trans fat, so don't buy it. Limit foodstuffs like cheese, whole milk, red meat and eggs, all of which are laden with cholesterol.

Whole grains promote heart health. Eat oats, brown rice and wholegrain bread. Adhere to the 'five a day' guideline for fruit and veg, as their fibres mop up fat. Choose fish over meat. If you insist on washing your meal down with alcohol, don't do it to excess as this increases fat levels. Some studies show that drinking one unit a day can increase HDL levels but the evidence is against excess alcohol.

Watch your weight as the greater your BMI (body mass index), the greater the potential burden of blood fat. Exercise for thirty minutes five days a week. The overall effect of exercise on your cholesterol, blood pressure and cardiovascular system cannot be overemphasised. And it goes without saying that you need to stop smoking.

Blood tests

Although a finger prick of blood can tell you what your cholesterol levels are, the gold standard is giving blood from a vein. Try to fast for between twelve and sixteen hours beforehand (you can have water though) as this will give a true picture of your cholesterol values. Americans advocate having a baseline cholesterol test at age twenty and then a test every five years. Remember that high cholesterol has no symptoms, so a blood sample is the only clue to unlocking your levels. Your doctor will also test your triglyceride levels – this is another type of fat, usually from food, that causes problems in excess.

Who should get tested? *You need a check-up if any of these applies to you:*

▌ Your dad or brother had a heart attack or heart disease before the age of fifty-five, or your mum or sister before the age of sixty-five

▌ You have high cholesterol or high blood pressure in the family

▌ You are over forty

▌ You have high blood pressure or diabetes

▌ You are overweight.

Who needs pills?

If diet and exercise fail to shift the fat burden and you're in a high-risk category for complications, you may need pills. Unfortunately, in the context of cholesterol, even your best effort is sometimes not good enough to get it down. Cholesterol-lowering medication saves lives, but treatment has to be lifelong – if you stop it, your cholesterol goes straight back up again.

Prescriptions Tests need to be done before you can start cholesterol treatment to check your pre-treatment cholesterol levels and liver function. The treatments used are called statins, and they work by reducing cholesterol production in the liver. However, they can have side-effects such as aches and pains, insomnia and indigestion. Your doctor will monitor your progress to work out the dose most suitable for you and check your blood for any evidence of side-effects on the liver or muscles. If you cannot tolerate statins, there are other options, so talk to your doctor.

Tips ▌ *Choosing to stop cholesterol pills without medical advice may be the choice between life and death. One in seven women in Europe die from coronary heart disease – don't become a statistic just because you can't be bothered to take a tablet.*

▌ *And don't assume your blood pressure is fine – let the doctor decide by checking it.*

Myth ▌ *You can eat what you like when you are on cholesterol pills. No you can't – eating the wrong foods can undo all the good effects of your medication.*

GOOD FAT / BAD FAT FOR NATURAL CHOLESTEROL MANAGEMENT

Dietary fat / cholesterol	Main source	State at room temperature	Effect on cholesterol levels	% of daily calorie intake*
Total fat				20%–35% (60–85g)
Monounsaturated fat – better	Olive oil, Canola oil, peanut oil, walnuts, almonds, peanuts, most other nuts, avocados, olives	Liquid	Lowers LDL No change in HDL	Up to 20% (49g)
Polyunsaturated fat – good	Corn, soybean, safflower and cottonseed oils; fish	Liquid	Lowers LDL Lowers HDL	Up to 10% (25g)
Saturated fat – bad	Whole milk, butter, cheese, and ice cream; red meat; chocolate; coconuts, coconut oil	Solid	Raises both LDL and HDL	Limit to no more than 7% (16g)
Trans fat – worst	Most margarines; vegetable shortening; partially hydrogenated vegetable oil; many processed foods	Solid or semi-solid	Raises LDL Lowers HDL	0 Allowance specified Keep at low levels
Cholesterol– bad but not as bad as saturated fat and trans fat	Eggs, non- skimmed dairy, fatty red meat	N/A	Raises LDL Raises HDL	Limit to no more than 200mg

grams in a 2200 calorie diet

PALPITATIONS

We define a palpitation as an awareness of the heart beat – fast, slow, missed or erratic. Generally, our heart beats away and, just like our breathing, we can't live without this, even though we are usually blissfully unaware of it. Doctors use the term arrhythmia to define an abnormal heart beat. Although we classically think of pacemakers being in the domain of the elderly, we all have a little electrical node in the muscle of our heart that acts like these to set the pace of our heart beat. When it decides not to work, that's when it is replaced by an artificial pacemaker.

What causes palpitations?

Most of us have the occasional irregular beat, and by and large the irregular thumps tend to be benign, but on occasion arrhythmias can be serious and sometimes life-threatening. We define a fast heart beat as over one hundred beats per minute and term this a tachycardia. This occurs with fever, exercise, stimulants such as caffeine or thyroid problems, and often for no apparent reason.

A slow heart beat is called bradycardia, and we use that term for anything below sixty beats per minute. This can occur if you are very fit, have a thyroid problem or have a problem with your pacemaker.

Problem beats

If your heart is beating very quickly and is irregular, this may be a sign of a serious underlying problem. The most common type of this is called atrial fibrillation; this is where the heart beats quickly in an irregular fashion and beats a lot faster than the pulse. This is a serious condition and can increase your risk of stroke.

Many other rhythms, both fast and slow, can also result in a variety of symptoms other than palpitations. Dizziness, chest pain, sweating, fainting, shortness of breath or light-headedness can all occur. It is possible, however, that you make feel nothing from an abnormal beat, hence the importance of feeling the beat, i.e. taking the pulse.

Taking your pulse

This is easy. Place two fingers on the thumb side of the wrist and you will feel your pulse ripple under your fingers. Count the number of beats that occur in fifteen seconds and multiply by four – this gives you your number of beats per minute. If you are not fit and this figure is under sixty, your heart may be too slow. If the beat is over a hundred or if it feels irregular or erratic, this could be the first sign of a problem with the electrics in your heart. In either of these cases, go and see your doctor for a check-up.

Is there a problem?

In young fit adults, there is often no serious problem, but many young women become very aware of their heart beat late at night in bed. You doctor will advise some blood tests, a heart tracing (known as an ECG or EKG) and twenty-four-hour monitoring that monitors your heart beat throughout the day and night. There is often nothing serious detected, and it is simply a question of eliminating things that can trigger the problem.

TAKING YOUR PULSE

Place two fingers on the thumb side of the wrist and you will feel your pulse ripple under your fingers.

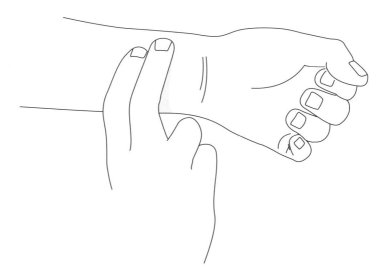

What affects the beat?

- Tea, coffee and cola – these all stimulate the heart
- Cocaine and amphetamines
- Cigarettes
- Alcohol
- Spicy foods

- Stimulants in cough and cold medicines
- Menopause
- Lack of magnesium in the diet
- Diet pills
- Food colourants and preservatives.

Treatments If nothing sinister is detected, there is nothing further to do. Medication may be needed for certain types of abnormal rhythm. If this doesn't work, the heart sometimes needs to be 'shocked' to reset the heart beat. If this fails, keyhole surgery may be needed to work on the electrics in the heart; alternatively, an artificial pacemaker may need to be inserted.

Common sense

If you find that any food stuff or activity gives you palpitations, give it up. This doesn't mean giving up exercise though as that's meant to make your heart beat faster! Don't use simple palpitations as an excuse not to exercise.

Have a look at your lifestyle. If stress, alcohol and coffee play a big role, remove them. Magnesium levels in the diet become depleted from too much caffeine and also dip in the menopause. This can be a factor in palpitations, but an adequate amount can be ingested by ditching coffee and eating a portion of raw broccoli a day. If you don't fancy that, two bananas will also work the magic on your magnesium levels!

Tip *Tell the doctor about all your recreational habits – the good, the bad and the ugly – as this is likely to provide a key to the cause.*

Myth *Diet pills are safe, and doctors are just scare-mongering over them. Wrong. Munch them at your peril as they can cause palpitations.*

CHEST PAINS

Could I be having a heart attack?

Yes is the answer. Whenever a patient describes a pain in their chest, alarm bells ring in both the patient's and doctor's head. Heart disease is very rare in menstruating women, and by and large you are less liable to suffer a heart attack until you hit the menopause. We generally label chest pain as cardiac or non-cardiac.

When should I act?

Don't ignore severe crushing squeezing pain or pressure in the chest if it lasts for more than a few minutes. Other warning signs are if it moves to the jaw or down the arm and you feel weak, sweaty or clammy. Don't waste time – dial for the emergency services. This could be a heart attack (where the blood supply to the heart becomes blocked, resulting in damage to the heart muscle) or angina, in which the blood supply to the heart becomes interrupted. As a woman, you are more likely to suffer from this if you have a family history of heart disease, you smoke, you have high blood pressure or cholesterol, you suffer from diabetes or you have had the menopause.

What if it's not my heart?

The younger you are, the less likely it is to be your heart, but that doesn't mean it's not serious. Chest pain and shortness of breath may be the sign of a lung clot. This can occur in women on the oral contraceptive pill, after an operation, after a long-haul flight, in overweight smokers or with any permutation of these. It can kill you if it goes unchecked. Pericarditis, which is inflammation of the heart muscle, can also be a reason, and this can come on after a virus, giving rise to severe chest pain.

Lung problems Tightness of the airways can result in chest pain. This can happen to susceptible people – with asthma or allergies – after exercise or exposure to lung irritants. Pleurisy – inflammation of the covering surrounding the lung – can produce chest pain, and this is often accompanied by fever. A pneumothorax or collapsed lung will give rise to chest pain of sudden onset with associated shortness of breath.

Gut problems Acid reflux and ulcers can cause chest pain. This very often comes on at 3am when acid production is at its maximum. A night on the tiles can result in chest pain due to gastritis (inflammation of the stomach lining).

Joints Your skeleton can be implicated too, whereby any problem such as wear and tear or inflammation in the chest wall cavity can produce pain. This pain can often be reproduced by touching the area. Tietze's syndrome is the name given to inflammation in the costal cartilages. It is also called costochondritis and generally occurs in the region of the second or third rib, with pain being felt where the rib joins the breast bone. It is most common in young adults who are physically active.

The gym Overactivity may cause muscular strain, so anything from an intense aerobic session to strenuous gardening may result in a strained muscle in the chest cavity that can cause pain.

Your job Stress and anxiety can cause chest tightness and discomfort. This leads to further worry that you may have a heart problem, so is self-perpetuating.

Cocaine Emergency departments see many patients after they have taken cocaine. Because it constricts the blood vessels, it can both cause chest pain and have serious cardiac consequences such as heart attacks.

What the doctor will do?

You doctor will take note of the nature of your pain. Say how long it stays there, what brings it on, what relieves it and whether there are any associated symptoms such as belching or sweating. No matter how stupid your symptom sounds, we need to know. You will have a general examination, a blood pressure measurement and probably an ECG (EKG) – a trace of the heart's electric activity that shows how healthy your heart is. If your doctor is worried, he or she will send you straight to the emergency department for tests. If this is the drill, don't drive, and don't defer going because you're about to have an important meeting – it could be the difference between life and death. If you don't need emergency treatment, you are likely to need blood tests, maybe a treadmill test and a chest X-ray depending on what the doctor believes the culprit is.

VARICOSE VEINS

I have these; I inherited them from my mother, who in turn inherited them from her father! They are easy to self-diagnose because they tend to make your veins look lumpy, protruding and tortuous. They generally crop up on the legs and, sorry to be the bearer of bad news, but 30 per cent of ladies develop them during their lifetime. We are twice as likely to suffer as men.

But the good news

Although they are ugly and can be uncomfortable, varicose veins are not usually that serious. Many women are happy to hide them away under their opaque tights and only opt for treatment if they become uncomfortable, unsightly or if they develop other problems such as leg ulcers or dermatitis. If you are planning to fall pregnant, it is best to postpone any procedure on the veins until you have completed your family.

Why do they occur?

Blood is delivered from your heart down to your legs via your arteries, and then back to your heart via your veins. This involves the blood having to flow upwards from the legs to the heart, so we use our muscles to push it up against gravity. Blood from the outer layers of your legs is transported through the superficial veins, and that from the deeper layers through the deep veins. All of these veins have valves to ensure that the flow goes in one direction only. If the valves stop working, there is a back-flow of blood and an increase in pressure, particularly when standing. This causes the veins to swell and the blood to pool, resulting in the bulges and twists in the veins that we can see on our lower limbs.

What makes them more likely?

Pregnancy is a factor, and they tend to crop up in the first trimester. If you are lucky, however, they will disappear three months after delivery. Varicose veins also tend to run in families. Prolonged standing doesn't help, and same is true for excess weight and immobility.

What are the possible problems?

Let's face it, they're ugly. But they can also be itchy and result in a dermatitis forming over the vein. If you get a cut in the area, it may take a long time to heal, and people with poor immunity or the elderly may develop an ulcer. Skin discoloration may occur, in particular around the ankle, where it can take on a rusty brown hue. Sometimes the vein becomes inflamed. We call this phlebitis, and it results in the vein becoming red, hard and painful. Luckily, it's easily treated by your family doctor.

Tests If you decide to have treatment for your veins, you will be seen by a vascular surgeon. The surgeon will use a procedure called a Doppler scan to detect the blood flow in the veins. Ultrasound is also used to work out where the flow problem is.

Treatments The visible appearance of the varicose veins tends to prove more of a problem in women than the actual vein itself. If treatment is necessary, the affected vein can be stripped away under anaesthetic. Another treatment is called sclerotherapy; this involves squirting a chemical into the vein that damages it, causing it to close up. This is done while you are awake. Laser therapy and electric currents applied directly to the vein can achieve a similar result by damaging the vein and causing it to close up.

Self-help

Watch your weight, and if you are sitting or standing in one position try to move around every thirty minutes. Compression stockings, although unfashionable, can control symptoms and prevent skin complications. Make sure you get measured up for the right size and be consistent about wearing them.

POOR CIRCULATION

Is poor circulation causing my fingers to go blue?

Raynaud's phenomenon is a condition affecting the circulation in the blood vessels supplying skin. It occurs when the tiny blood vessels supplying the skin of the fingers and feet become constricted in response to heat, cold or other stimuli.

Poor circulation means it's most likely in old ladies, right?

No, this is a very common condition that can occur at all ages, but it's much more common in women. It is estimated that one in twenty of the population suffers from it, and about 10 per cent of women in the UK have it to some degree. You might first notice it in the winter months, beginning in your teens and twenties – your fingers go icy cold and turn white. Sometimes they then turn blue, and then because the vessels open up again, they get a surge of blood and turn red. Accompanying this, you get numbness, tingling and pain. It's generally the hands that are ravaged by Raynaud's, occasionally the feet and less so the nose, ear lobes or even the nipples or tongue.

Is it dangerous?

In 90 per cent of cases, Raynaud's is not a sign of any underlying problem with the circulation. It implies that the tiny blood vessels supplying your skin are oversensitive. In this most common form, Raynaud's does not usually cause any mischief, although it can be the source of a lot of annoyance.

In about one in ten cases, Raynaud's is the sign of an underlying disease such as lupus. In this instance, the symptoms will usually start later, so the first sign of a circulatory problem may not be until the thirties. The form of Raynaud's associated with another disease tends to follow the path of that disorder and may lead to gangrene and ulcers of the affected areas due to severe problems with the circulation.

Can Raynaud's be treated?

A drug called nifedipine can sometimes be used. This opens up blood vessels, and by improving the circulation it improves the symptoms. Because it opens up all the blood vessels and not just the ones affected by Raynaud's, it causes dizziness, headache and flushing in 75 per cent of those who take it, so the treatment may prove worse than the disorder. Other blood pressure drugs such as ACE inhibitors and calcium channel blockers have also been tried, but the response is very individual. With any drug, you should try them for at least a fortnight as you often become tolerant to their side-effects.

Remember that medications aren't a cure, and you still need to wrap up. Ideally, taking precautions to prevent exposure to extreme cold or heat is the best bet. Glove up, and do so indoors as well if you need to. Keep the whole body and not just the affected areas warm. You can buy mini heat packs if your symptoms are very severe. Avoid getting food out of the freezer or de-icing the car in the mornings. Stop smoking and exercise more, both of which improve blood flow.

Too cold for comfort?

Although this condition is common, see your doctor if you feel your symptoms are excessive and you really can't warm up. Make a diary of your symptoms and the specific temperatures and activities that are affected. Mention any female relatives similarly affected, both past and present. Also let the doctor know of any family history of rheumatoid arthritis, lupus or other joint disorders. Your doctor will order blood tests and may refer you to a specialist if they feel your problem is due to an underlying disease.

Tips ▌ *If your hands need a quick warm-up, immerse them in warm water.*

▌ *Smoking outdoors can reduce your body temperature by one degree centigrade for a full twenty minutes. So stop smoking or suffer!*

Lungs

5

These are the most important airbags you will ever be issued with. Learn about what can go wrong with our ventilation system and how to act if there's a problem.

ACHOO OR THE FLU?

On average we catch two to five colds a year. Autumn and winter are the busiest seasons for bugs. Over two hundred virus types can cause the 'common' cold, but rhinoviruses are the winners. These cook best at 33°C (91°F), which is the ambient temperature in the nose, so no wonder they prosper. Other likely candidates are coronavirus, adenovirus and the influenza virus.

So how do you catch a cold or flu? Science suggests these bugs grow best in autumn and winter temperatures, and as we tend to cluster indoors when the temperature drops, we provide an environment in which they party. Physical and psychological stress are also implicated as they lower our immune response to infection.

To physically 'catch' a cold or flu, you need to inhale infected mucus or touch an infected surface and then touch your mouth, nose or eyes. Beware – a simple sneeze can contain up to one hundred thousand virus particles and can travel nine metres (thirty feet). In turn, these little particles can live on both the skin surface or the surface of an object for up to three hours.

So do I have a cold or a flu?

Chances are that if you have a fever of 38°C (100°F) or more, sweats, aches and pains, a headache, a dry cough, a sore throat and fatigue, you probably have flu. You feel jet lagged, and you wouldn't look twice at an attractive man on the bus. On the other hand, if you feel bunged up and very sorry for yourself, you are likely to have what one billion Americans suffer from annually… a cold.

If it really is the flu, stay home, drink lots of non-alcoholic fluids, ditch the diet, eat carbohydrates and bin the gym; rest is the best medicine. Take simple analgesia such as paracetamol or ibuprofen for aches and fevers – it's safe to take them together, but always read the label and never exceed the daily dose no matter how desperate you feel. And remember that antibiotics won't help as they don't work for viruses.

The seasonal flu vaccine helps to prevent flu in 70 to 90 per cent of cases and is a must if you have a condition that lowers your immunity. The jab takes about two weeks to become fully functional.

Tips
- *Invest in a hand sanitiser and keep those paws clean.*
- *Wipe down communal areas with antiviral/antibacterial wipes.*
- *Buy tissues, use them, offer them to other sufferers on the train and remember to bin them rather than just leaving them in your handbag.*
- *If you find yourself in a crowded area and you haven't got a tissue, sneeze or cough into your elbow; you are far less likely to cross-infect anyone.*
- *Eat healthily, take lots of exercise and sleep – it's the best medicine. Zinc, vitamin C, echinacea, cod liver oil and honey are all cited as being helpful. Science is somewhat in dispute about this, but one thing is for sure, they do no harm.*

Swine flu

2009 saw swine flu strike with a vengeance, and we went from an outbreak to an epidemic – a large collection of cases in a locality – to a pandemic, where a disease is widespread across a country or a continent. Just like regular flu, swine flu proved to be very contagious and without cure.

Antiviral treatments such as oseltamivir (Tamiflu) were given in an effort to alleviate symptoms and in many cases shorten the illness by one to two days. Although these drugs have not been proven to prevent flu, they are sometimes given to people who have been in contact with the virus to improve their defences. An inhaled antiviral agent called zanamivir (Relenza) can be used for pregnant women as oseltamivir may damage the unborn baby.

Because these drugs have been used on a widespread basis, there have been concerns that swine flu could become resistant to them and render them useless. For this reason, they should not be taken unless it's pretty certain you have swine flu. The doctor can diagnose it by means of a swab, but the results are not instant, so the decision of whether to treat often has to be made on the spot during the consultation.

To vaccinate or not?

Anyone can get flu, but those over sixty-five and those with other illnesses such as diabetes, asthma or heart disease are more at risk and should have the shot. Most of my patients who do not want the vaccine say it's because it 'gave them the flu last year'. But that's not true – it's a dead vaccine made up of inactivated flu virus so you can't catch flu. Some people do get flu-like symptoms forty-eight hours later, but that's their immune system reacting to the vaccine. It takes about seven to ten days for you to be deemed immune after the shot. The vaccination contains some antibiotics, and one brand of the vaccine has been manufactured in hens eggs so is unsuitable if you have an egg allergy.

Swine flu vaccine essentially operates on the same premise as standard flu vaccine, i.e. it's dead and delivered via the same medium. Pregnant women are a specific risk group for swine flu, and studies show the vaccine is not harmful to the unborn baby. The consequences of swine flu in pregnancy can be serious and potentially fatal to both you and your unborn baby. So before you decide you don't want the vaccine, speak to your doctor.

Tip *Don't underestimate the flu – its complications can kill.*

Myth *The flu vaccine gives you the flu. No – it can't because the virus in the vaccine is dead.*

WHEN IS A COUGH A CHEST INFECTION?

THE LUNGS

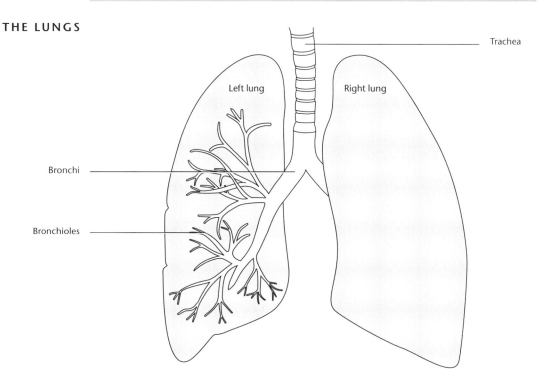

We get between two and four respiratory infections, referring to coughs and colds, each year. If everybody affected took antibiotics for each episode, the whole population would be on them for at least one month a year, assuming that we got about four infections a year each lasting a total seven days. These infections are usually caused by a virus, which means that antibiotics do not have any effect whatsoever, so if you are pill-taking you are time-wasting.

What might be a sign that I need to see a doctor?

The following are warning signs:

▐ If you are coughing up green gunk

▐ If you have coughed up any blood-stained or rusty spit

- If you feel tight in the chest or wheezy
- If you have sweats and a high fever
- If the cough has been going on for more than two weeks.

So I've got a simple cough; how do I sort it?

The most practical thing to do to tackle the tickle is rest, eat healthily and drinks lots of fluids. See your pharmacist to treat the symptoms of the cough – he or she will advise you on the best cough medicine as these vary for dry coughs, phlegmy coughs, etc. Aches and pains can be helped by simple painkillers like paracetamol and ibuprofen. Most importantly, be like the hospital Matron in the maintenance of your hand hygiene and handkerchiefs as failure to do so will not only spread the bugs, but is also likely to slow your recovery or spread the virus elsewhere, such as to your eyes.

What exactly is a chest infection?

We all have two lungs, and broadly speaking we refer to a 'chest infection' as any infection in the tubes going into the lungs or in the lungs themselves. Bronchitis occurs where the infection is in the tubes going into the lungs, which are known as the bronchi. Pneumonia occurs when the infection is in the lung tissue itself. It's called double pneumonia when it's in both lungs. However, fewer than one in a hundred of us will have pneumonia if we have the symptoms of a chest infection.

Bronchitis

This is really common in winter time and often affects smokers. It is usually, but not exclusively, caused by a virus, so when you see your doctor he or she may say that antibiotics are not needed and advise you that the bronchitis will disappear of its own accord in seven to ten days.

Pneumonia

Pneumonia tends to be caused by bacteria that you pick up when you are out and about. You feel more ill than with bronchitis and are unlikely to have any appetite or energy. You often sweat and feel weak.

Because pneumonia is usually caused by bacteria, it is normally treated with antibiotics. Although most pneumonia is caused specifically by the pneumonia bacterium (*Streptococcus pneumoniae*), it can be caused by others as well. It is possible to vaccinate against this, and it is now part of the childhood immunisation programme in the UK, Ireland, USA and Australia. The elderly and high-risk groups are also offered the vaccination.

Pneumonia generally takes longer to get over than bronchitis, so don't expect to be back at work for at least two weeks. And remember that severe pneumonia may need to be treated in hospital.

So what's pleurisy?

This is an inflammation of the 'skin' lining the lung. The lung is covered by two layers of membrane called pleurae, one surrounding the lung and the other lining the chest cavity. There is some fluid in between the two layers to help prevent friction when the lungs inflate. If this lining gets inflamed, it's called pleurisy, and this usually happens after an infection. Pleurisy results in a pain when you breathe in or out, shortness of breath and a dry cough. As it is often due to a virus, it is treated with anti-inflammatories to kill the pain rather than antibiotics.

Tips *Get your doctor to check that you are fit before going back to work after pneumonia – rushing back may result in you relapsing.*

Persisting symptoms forty-eight hours into taking antibiotics warrants a further review – if they are the appropriate treatment, they really should have kicked in by now.

Myth *Antibiotics are essential for all chest infections. No they aren't, as many chest infections are due to a virus.*

WHEN IS A COUGH ASTHMA?

One in twelve adults suffer from asthma, which often starts in childhood. More women than men, however, develop it in adulthood. If your doctor tells you have asthma, don't despair – although it isn't curable, it is manageable. Although we commonly associate asthma with wheezing, the presenting symptom is often a cough.

What is asthma anyway?

Asthma happens when a trigger such as dust irritates the airways and causes the muscles to tighten, so the air pipe is squeezed inwards, and in turn its lining becomes inflamed and swells, narrowing it further. That's why you get wheezing as the air flows in against resistance, hence the noise. It's a bit like sucking air in through a straw.

So who is more likely to suffer from asthma?

You can tick the box if you fit into any of the following: you have hay fever or allergy, you have eczema, you're overweight, you're a smoker or you have a family history of asthma.

What are the symptoms?

You may notice a wheeze, a cough, shortness of breath and a tight chest.

What makes the symptoms worse?

- A cough or cold
- Exercise
- Cigarette smoke
- A change in temperature
- Pollutants at work or home, such as air conditioning and animals
- Early morning or late at night as that's when our airways naturally 'sleep'.

How can a cough be asthma?

Your cough could actually be the symptom of your airways narrowing, which can make you cough, wheeze, gasp for breath or feel tight in the chest. So although a wheeze is the symptom we are all familiar with, not every asthmatic wheezes.

How is it diagnosed?

It's often a clinical diagnosis made by the doctor based on your history and an examination. The doctor may ask you to blow into a peak flow meter, which measures how fast the air is coming out of your lungs. This is then compared with the average for your age, height and sex. If the diagnosis is in doubt, spirometry (a set of breathing tests) is carried out to confirm the diagnosis.

Are you an asthmatic forever?

The propensity for asthma will always remain, but that does not mean that you will always need treatment.

How do you help it?

If your asthma is mild, you will simply have a pump to use as needed when you have symptoms. This is commonly called the 'reliever'. This is a quick fix and widens up your wind pipes in a matter of minutes.

If you have to use this frequently, for example more than three times a week, you wake with asthma in the night or you get symptoms such as the ones listed above, you need a steroid inhaler. Don't panic about the steroid inhaler – you won't beef up or grow a beard using it. The aim here is to deliver the steroid to where it is needed, i.e. just the lung and not elsewhere. The difference between the steroid inhaler and the other inhaler, the pump, is that the steroid inhaler takes longer to act, so it is usually a week or more before you see its value. Be patient.

Tablets can also be used to dampen down the allergic response and help open up the airways, but inhalers are generally the first line of attack. An acute bout of asthma is often treated with steroid tablets for five to ten days. These generally provide immense relief but are no substitute for regular management as they have significant side-effects.

Helping your asthma

- Don't smoke.
- Know what triggers your asthma.
- Do regular exercise.

▌ If exercise triggers your asthma, take a few puffs of your reliever inhaler twenty minutes before you play sport and again afterwards.

Get shown how to use your inhalers – so many patients squirt the medicine into the sky and not into their lungs. There are lots of different designs of device to help get the drugs to where they are needed. And if you aren't making progress, don't give up. Instead, go back to the doctor as they need to know you are having difficulty. Know when your tubes are suffering and make sure you have an emergency action plan for attacks. Also make sure you get the flu jab each winter if you have chronic asthma. And finally, if you use a steroid inhaler, rinse your mouth out after using it to prevent oral thrush.

Think you might have asthma?

Asthma can be very mild and is not always accompanied by a wheeze. So see your doctor for a check of your lungs and a chat about your symptoms. You may need a chest X-ray or some blood tests. The diagnosis is usually straightforward and made in the doctor's office. A lingering cough is sometimes a symptom of asthma so get it checked out.

Tips ▌ *If your asthma is triggered by exercise, cold or emotion, don't dive – it could trigger an attack.*

▌ *Inhalers normally contain one hundred and twenty doses, but just like a can of deodorant they can be empty when you badly need them. So if you have more than one handbag, make sure you have more than one inhaler. Asthma doesn't necessarily accompany a particular outfit, so you could 'go without' by mistake.*

Ears, nose and throat

6

From snoring to sore throats and popping ears, learn more about everything ENT.

SORE THROAT

YOUR THROAT

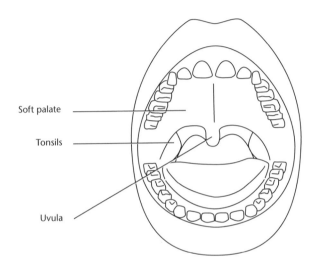

Soft palate

Tonsils

Uvula

Sore throat is an incredibly common symptom – we've all had one. We call a sore throat tonsillitis when the tonsils are the trouble and pharyngitis when it's the pharynx. Look at the diagram and you'll get an idea of which bit is which. Most infections are caused by a virus and tend to pass off after a few days. Paracetamol and ibuprofen help to ease the pain. The old wives' tale of drinking plenty and getting lots of rest holds true here. It also helps to gargle with soluble aspirin in lukewarm water for about three minutes, repeated four times a day. Remember though that aspirin is not suitable for everyone.

What about antibiotics?

Antibiotics are usually not necessary as most infections are caused by viruses, and antibiotics don't work on viral infections. And even if the sore throat is due to a mild bacterial infection, you can usually fight it yourself. So the doctor isn't trying to be awkward by saying no – it makes sense not to sign up to a week of antibiotics when you can usually cure yourself in a couple of days.

So when should I go to the doctor?

If you have a very severe sore throat or tonsillitis with a high fever or feel very unwell and have a rash, see your doctor. If your sore throat is lingering for more than four days

113

or seems different from previous attacks, get a check. And if you have any difficulty in swallowing or breathing, it goes without saying that you should seek advice.

What else could it be?

A streptococcal throat infection causes pus covered tonsils, fever and sometimes a rash, and can lead to complications. It's often termed 'strep throat' and is contagious; it requires ten days' antibiotics to kill the bacteria. Glandular fever is due to a virus and often starts with a sore throat. A postnasal drip from a sinus problem and acid reflux can both cause symptoms. If you have oral thrush, your throat will be both sore and taste bad. Remember that if you smoke and suffer a sore throat for longer than two weeks, it could be the first sign of a more sinister problem, so get it seen.

Should I have my tonsils out?

Adult patients often ask this. We don't usually encourage adults to have their tonsils out unless it is totally necessary, which I would define as more than six episodes of severe tonsillitis in the last year requiring antibiotics and time off work. The tonsils can be removed by surgery, zapped with laser or given heat treatment. The doctor tries to put you off having your tonsils out because the risk of bleeding after a tonsillectomy is much greater in an adult than in a child – five out of every hundred adults who have their tonsils out end up returning to hospital due to haemorrhage. Don't rush into a tonsillectomy unless it is your only way out of tonsil hell. It will require about ten days to two weeks off work and at least one night in hospital.

What's quinsy?

Quinsy is an abscess forming around the tonsil as a consequence of tonsillitis. It's incredibly painful and results in a very high temperature and difficulty in swallowing. You'd be unlucky to get this once; get it twice and your local ENT surgeon will advise that you have your tonsils out as it is a sign that it could keep coming back.

Tip   *Sore throat and recent unprotected sexual activity may be the first symptoms of gonorrhoea.*

STUFFED-UP SINUSES

No one is exactly sure what purpose our sinuses serve, but one thing's for sure, if they play up, it's a real pain for us. The sinuses are pockets of air lying in the skull that are connected to the nasal passages. There are four main sets of sinuses, lying behind the cheekbones, in the forehead, and next to the nose and the eyes. It's the ones in the cheeks that are the biggest and tend to cause the most mischief.

So what happens in sinusitis?

The lining of the sinus becomes inflamed. The mucus that is normally produced by this lining is usually drained through the nose, but if it builds up the sinus becomes waterlogged and transforms from a dry sponge to a wet sponge. This means that the mucus stagnates and becomes infected, and there is a build-up of pressure.

You will tend to feel pain and pressure in the affected area, usually below the eyes. You may also have a headache, a fever, a blocked nose and a thick, gunky, blood-stained nasal discharge. Sometimes your teeth will ache too.

What causes it?

▌ It can be due to a viral, a bacterial or rarely a fungal infection.

▌ A dental infection can also result in sinusitis.

▌ Patients with nasal allergies, nasal polyps or asthma are more susceptible, as are those whose nasal septum is deviated, which means that the bit dividing their nose in two is crooked. This can occur after breaking your nose.

▌ If you smoke, you are also more susceptible to sinus problems.

Can it be fixed?

Sinusitis is described as acute if it arrives quickly and disappears quickly. We term it chronic if it lingers for longer than three months. Acute, i.e. quick, sinusitis is generally caused by a virus and will not be helped by antibiotics. You can, however, take painkillers to ease the symptoms, antihistamines to dry up the mucus and a steroid nasal spray to help with the inflammation. Steam also helps to unblock the nose, but take care when doing this that you don't scald yourself.

If your symptoms persist or if you are worried, see your doctor as you may have developed a bacterial infection. This occurs in about one in three cases. In this instance, antibiotics will help, but they usually need to be taken for ten to fourteen days, so make sure you complete the course even if you feel better. And don't expect your doctor to send off any tests as X-rays, nose swabs and blood tests really don't aid in the diagnosis.

Lingering symptoms for over three months suggest a chronic problem. One minute you feel fine; the next the sinusitis is back with a bang. You may notice your breath becoming smelly, a runny nose, pressure in your face and a poor sense of smell. See your doctor, who can refer you to an ENT specialist if there is no obvious cause.

An ENT surgeon can put a telescope into your sinus and remove anything that is blocking the drainage system. The specialist can also remove any nasal polyps and straighten any anatomical abnormalities that might be hindering drainage. Remember that a visit to an ENT surgeon does not always mean an operation, and you may leave the consultation with a prescription for a nasal spray to be taken for three months, or a four week course of antibiotics.

Tip ▌ *Don't treat a chronic sinus problem with over-the-counter decongestant sprays. Not only will this not cure the problem, it will create another one by causing a constantly runny nose.*

HOARSENESS

Medics call hoarseness dysphonia, meaning a weak or altered voice or difficulty in making sounds. We make sounds by causing our vocal cords to vibrate, so anything that interferes with that process causes vocal problems.

So what stops the vocal cords vibrating properly?

Infections are the most common cause – laryngitis due to bacteria or a virus. Be warned – the strenuous use of the voice during a bout of laryngitis can cause long-term damage. So when the doctor says shut up, they really do mean shut up! Overuse, for example in telephonists, is the next most common cause. Sometimes you can also develop nodules on your vocal cords as a result of overuse, as seen in singers and teachers. Hoarseness can be the first sign of something sinister like a head, neck, lung or thyroid tumour if the cancer infiltrates the nerve to the voice box. General problems with nerves and muscles can also bring about hoarseness, and it can be the presenting symptom of a thyroid problem.

What contributes to it?

Smoking, any occupation in which the voice is overused, alcohol, acid reflux and nasal blockage.

Should I worry?

Anyone who has persistent hoarseness for longer than three weeks needs checking out. This is usually done by an ENT specialist who looks at the voice box with a device called a laryngoscope. This can be done while you are awake.

How can it be helped?

If it has been established that there is not an underlying problem, the following will all help. Stop cigarettes and alcohol. Control acid reflux, and keep hydrated. And if you feel you're getting hoarse, rest your voice. If problematic, singer's nodules can be removed under general anaesthetic. Vocal coaching by a speech therapist also helps.

Tip ▌ *Remember – persistent hoarseness for longer than three weeks must be checked out.*

117

GLANDULAR FEVER

There are lots of names for this condition. The Brits call it glandular fever (as your glands swell up), the Americans call it 'mono' (short for mononucleosis), and most medics refer to it as EBV (Epstein–Barr virus) after the chaps who discovered it. Haven't had it? Well, you may have had it but not have realised. It seems that over half of the adult population have some form of immunity to it, which probably developed when they were young.

What are the symptoms?

Glandular fever can start off with mild symptoms of headache and tiredness before the sore throat and fever begin to kick in. This is then accompanied by enlargement of the glands in the neck and often the armpits and groin as well.

This phase lasts one or two weeks. In some people, the liver can become inflamed, giving rise to what's called hepatitis. This in turn may result in jaundice, which can make your skin go yellow. In other people, the spleen can become enlarged. This organ sits tucked behind the rib cage on the left side of the body and serves to both break down and manufacture blood cells. We tend not to hear much about the spleen though unless it's giving us grief.

How is glandular fever contracted?

Yet another name for this illness is kissing disease. It is passed through saliva, which is why long lingering lunges could result in quarantine if you catch it. On a more mundane level though, it can also be spread by sharing drinking utensils or by coughing and sneezing, so don't worry, your doctor won't instantly think you have been in some passionate clinch! Glandular fever can take about six weeks to appear after you come into contact with it.

How do you diagnose it?

Your doctor can do a blood test, called a Monospot, to check whether you have glandular fever. The test can sometimes be negative early on and may need repeating if it seems likely that you have the disease. The levels of EBV antibodies can also be tested – high levels of IgM antibody (Ig stands for immunoglobulin) show that you currently have the infection, and high levels of IgG show that you have cleared it and are immune.

But antibiotics will get rid of it, won't they?

No, no, no! Basic biology here – this is a virus, and we know that antibiotics don't work against viruses, so they won't help here. This is another one of those conditions for which there is no cure. About 10 per cent of people have a co-existent bacterial infection in the throat and do require antibiotics, but for everyone else it's a case of self-management.

Steroids are occasionally prescribed in severe cases – they don't actually cure anything but they may ease the symptoms in certain situations. However, the evidence for their use still hangs in the balance.

So what do I do?

Stay home and expect to be there for at least two to four weeks. As glandular fever passes, you tend to feel profoundly tired, lethargic and often depressed. Make sure you drink lots of water, rest and eat healthily.

If you play contact sports, you need to avoid these until you get clearance from your doctor that your spleen has recovered – playing ladies' rugby with an enlarged spleen could kill you if your spleen ruptures. So you need to stay off the pitch for six to eight weeks.

Recovery

Most people are back in action between two and four weeks later. Others, however, take three to six months to get over the chronic fatigue that sometimes accompanies this illness, and there are a minor few who can take years to do so.

NOSEBLEEDS

As with many conditions, doctors aren't happy to call a nosebleed simply a nosebleed – we term it an epistaxis. Although this sounds like an exotic cocktail, it actually comes from the Greek meaning 'dripping from'. Although nosebleeds are common in children, usually brought on by picking their nose, adults also succumb. So just because you are over ten years of age, don't think you have said goodbye to the blood-stained hanky.

Who gets them in their later years?

They usually strike when you are approaching your fiftieth year, right up until you are an octogenarian. If you suffer from hay fever or sinus problems, you are more susceptible. If your blood pressure is high, you take medication such as aspirin or warfarin or you are prone to picking your nose, you may also fall prey to nosebleeds. In addition, recreational cocaine snorting and excessive alcohol consumption make bleeding more likely.

Why does it happen?

Because of its prominent position on the face, it's no surprise that trauma can cause nosebleeds. When the lining of the nose dries out and cracks, such as in the winter months, after a cold or if you are addicted to cocaine, it becomes vulnerable and can bleed. The nose has a vast network of blood vessels so, depending on the area affected, it may range from a small amount of bleeding to a severe haemorrhage. People with high blood pressure are particularly vulnerable as this puts extra pressure on the network of blood vessels.

How do I stop it from bleeding?

Pinch the soft parts of your nose between your thumb and your index finger with your other fingers pressed firmly against the bones of the face. Tilt your head slightly forward and keep squeezing your nose for five minutes. Apply a bag of frozen peas to your nose and cheek area if you can. The main mistake people make is that they tilt their head backwards and end up swallowing blood. They also tend to gently squeeze the tip of the nose as if they are politely avoiding a smell, which is useless.

What if it keeps flowing?

Keep doing the above routine at ten minute intervals. If you must cough or sneeze, do so with your mouth open to avoid a build-up of pressure. Straining on the toilet may start the bleeding off again, as may a soothing cup of tea or a cigarette after the event. Sit quietly with your head above the level of your heart.

If you are bleeding heavily, cannot stop the bleeding or feel faint, you should seek medical attention as your circulation can become compromised by heavy blood loss. Enlist the help of a friend to get you to the nearest emergency room if things seem to be getting out of control. You may need to have the bleeding stopped by cautery – burning the bleeding vessel to stop its flow – or it may also necessitate a nasal pack, which is shaped like a tampon and placed inside the nose to absorb the blood.

How can I prevent nosebleeds?

If you are disgusting enough to be a nose picker, ditch the habit. In terms of other habits, cocaine usage is traumatic to the nose, causing bleeding, congestion, a runny nose and eventually collapse of the nose because the drug eats away at the nasal bones. Individuals with blood pressure problems need to have regular checks as nosebleeds can occur if the pressure isn't controlled. Interestingly, the most common cause of nosebleeds is the drying out of the lining inside the nose. To prevent this, apply Vaseline to the inside of the nose. Irrigating your nose with a saline spray can also help.

When should I worry?

Most nosebleeds are harmless. However, a new onset of nosebleeds in adults warrants a check-up to rule out blood pressure problems or bleeding disorders.

SNORING

Does your better half snore? My dog Dinky does, and I have to confess that I myself snore quite badly! Snoring is caused by parts of the nose and throat vibrating when you breathe in and out. OK then, but why don't we snore all day? Well, at night the muscles that support these structures become relaxed and so tend to vibrate more. To add to this, lying on the back obstructs the airway so that air flow becomes more turbulent. And any part of your nose and throat system that's blocked will cause you to snore.

What kinds of thing block the system?

If you have a cough or a cold or even hay fever, you are more likely to breathe through your mouth and snore as a result. If you have polyps up your nose, these will block the flow of air. If you smoke, you are twice as likely to snore as your airways will get inflamed and blocked. And if you are overweight, this puts extra pressure on your airways. Alcohol and any muscle relaxants will further relax those muscles at night and may precipitate snoring. In addition, about 40 per cent of pregnant women snore during the third trimester.

So what's the problem if I snore?

First of all, it's a big problem for others and has even been cited as a reason for divorce.

Apart from its impact on others, it could also be the sign of a condition called sleep apnoea, in which the relaxed airway muscles actually stop you breathing for periods during the night and starve your body of oxygen. The snorer usually stops breathing for several seconds and then appears to recommence snoring again. At its simplest, this type of pattern causes sleepiness and irritability the following day as the sleep is so frequently disturbed at night. In the long term, it can be associated with high blood pressure, strokes and heart attacks.

So yes, snoring has far more serious consequences than getting a kick from your partner in the middle of the night. People with serious sleep apnoea can even be banned from driving as they fall asleep at the wheel, so it's no joke.

So how do you solve the problem?

- Don't drink alcohol late at night.
- Keep your weight down – the thicker the neck, the louder the snore.
- Sleep on your side or on your belly. To aid this, sew a tennis ball into the back of your pyjamas.
- Raise the head of your bed.

Keep the nasal passages clear by using saline spray, eucalyptus oil or a humidifier in the room. If your nose seems blocked, see your doctor. You could have polyps, the fleshy things that grow down the nose and obstruct it.

The nose itself could be askew, perhaps from a previous break. This means that the septum – the divider down the middle of the nose that dissolves in cocaine addicts – may not be straight and may be obstructing your breathing. Your soft palate could also be floppy. Or your tonsils may be large. All of these things are easily treatable with the knife of an ENT surgeon.

HAY FEVER AND RHINITIS

About twenty-five per cent of us suffer from hay fever. It's due to an allergy to pollen, which is a powder produced by flowers, plants and grass. Doctors call it seasonal allergic rhinitis because different pollens are high during different seasons.

So why all the sneezing, wheezing and eye watering?

The menacing symptoms are due to histamine, which our immune system releases in response to something we are allergic to. The problem is that histamine can cause eyes to water, noses to run and sneeze, and sometimes lungs to wheeze and hives to erupt. Every bit of you that is physically exposed to the allergen can react.

Could I have hay fever?

Yes, your chances could be as high as one in four. Classically, it will result in spasms of sneezing and a runny nose. Unlike a cold, your nasal secretions will be free of bugs and you won't have a fever, but your nose may become blocked and your chest tight or wheezy. You're unlikely to produce any muck when you cough, but you're likely to have an irritating dry cough. Your eyes will water and look bloodshot, and constantly rubbing them will result in them getting puffy so you look like you are lacking sleep. But they shouldn't stick together like they would in an infection.

Who gets it?

First and foremost, you can't catch hay fever. It tends to run in families though and is often linked with asthma, eczema and allergy.

What should I do?

Work out which pollen pesters you and track its levels, either online or via the weather forecast. Some sites have a facility to alert you when the offending allergen is on the increase – you may be able to get a message sent to your mobile phone to warn you. A pollen count greater than fifty is considered high. Think silver birch, ash and oak if your symptoms occur in early spring, and grass pollen from spring to high summer – timothy grass is the worst offender. And think weeds and nettles at summer's end. Pre-empt your sneezing season by starting your treatment before the pollen starts on you.

Self-help Get a pair of sunglasses as they will protect your eyes. Buy big and buy wraparound. Vaseline smeared on the inside of the nose helps to trap pollen. It's a good idea to wash your hair and have a shower at the end of every day. Remember that the pollen count is low between 11am and 3pm, when the sun is at its highest – this is the best time to go out. And keep your car and bedroom windows closed during your sneezy season.

Which medication? Tackle the nose with an antihistamine and/or a steroid spray. The antihistamine spray generally works in about twenty minutes. It blasts the itch, watering and sneezing. Steroid sprays take longer to kick in – maybe a couple of days before you see a response. They do a similar job and also help unblock a clogged nose. Rather cleverly, they seem to have some effect on eye symptoms too. Beware buying a decongestant spray (the type used for sinus congestion) over the counter as using it for longer than five days may actually worsen your congestion.

Eyes Antihistamine drops have a quick effect on the eyes so are a must for the handbag. Cromoglicate (cromolyn) drops work well too but not as quickly. Both nasal steroids and antihistamine tablets also help with eye symptoms, so it may not be necessary to use multiple products. Antihistamine tablets can work like magic, affecting the nose, eyes and chest. Some make you drowsy, but the newer brands are generally well tolerated.

In dire straits? Doctors sometimes prescribe a course of steroid tablets to get you through important periods such as exams or a wedding. Because of the long-term side effects of steroids, however, this is only used as a last resort. It's no longer common practice to give steroid injections before the start of the season because of their long-term side-effects, for example, osteoporosis, muscle damage and cataracts. We also now have an excellent army of antihistamines that are just as effective.

Montelukast This was initially marketed for asthma sufferers but now has a licence for seasonal rhinitis. It acts by blocking leukotrienes, chemicals in the bloodstream that form part of the reaction in hay fever.

Desensitisation This is done by an immunologist or allergy specialist in a specialist clinic. Serial injections of pollen are given and the immune system gradually becomes desensitised to it. It's a bit like getting used to working with an obnoxious male colleague.

Tips
- *Have your hay fever response unit ready to spring into action just before the season hits.*
- *If you are pregnant, it's safe to use nasal steroid sprays and cromoglicate-based inhalers and eye drops, but best to avoid antihistamines.*

Hay fever when there isn't any hay?

If your beak is constantly blocked, sneezy, itchy or runny, you probably have perennial rhinitis. This is usually caused by allergens or irritants and leaves you with symptoms all year. You may actually be allergic to your home!

How clean is your house? House dust mite is ever present. We can't see it, but it drinks our sweat and eats our skin scales, and its faecal matter is the menace resulting in persistent rhinitis. Our pets can be a pest too. Their saliva and dead skin cells can cause allergy. And is there mould lurking in the shower or behind the fridge? You could be allergic to its spores – clean out your fridge and replace the earth in your indoor plants every 6 months. It goes without saying that allergy-proof bedding should be used and washed at 60°C. Get rid of carpets, and invest in a high-filter vacuum cleaner. Don't forget to use it on drapes and soft furnishings.

Tests It is often possible to identify the allergen and take measures to avoid it. If you are struggling, see your family doctor for allergy testing. This may be by a blood test to check the amount of IgE antibody you have in your bloodstream – the higher the level in response to a specific substance, the more allergic you are to it. The results are scored from one to six, six being the worst. Your doctor might also refer you for skin prick tests or patch tests, in which substances you may be allergic to are placed onto your skin and your reaction is monitored.

My doctor won't test me! If you draw a blank, you can have some allergy testing done though pharmacies. You can, for example, test for the ten most common inhaled allergies by using a fingerprick of blood on a device like a pregnancy test. The results are available in twenty minutes. Take care spending lots of money on other testing such as kinesiology, hair analysis or Vega testing. Doctors don't regard these as valid and they cannot verify a true allergy.

Treatment Persistent rhinitis and hay fever are managed in the same way. It's sensible to avoid triggers – which can include stress – so if you think you may be allergic to work, you may be right. Air conditioning or dust is often the cause and you'll find that your symptoms are better at the weekends. Do some detective work in the form of a diary.

Tip   *Recurrent use of nasal decongestants can actually cause persistent rhinitis, so beware – don't use them for longer than one week.*

Myth   *The dog has to go. No – in fact cats are the worst culprits. Wash your pets twice weekly if possible and groom them. Vacuum where they have been on a regular basis. Maximise your medical treatment and cleaning methods and you may find that Felix or Fido can stay.*

EARWAX

'Yuk'… 'Never put anything smaller than your elbow into your ear'… 'Wash your ears out'… 'What the heck is this stuff?' Well, ear wax is a protective coating over the skin in the ear that helps to clean and lubricate. It traps dirt, water and bacteria. It's horrid, but we need it or our ear skin will become dry and irritated.

Who suffers from ear wax?

Everyone with ears has ear wax, but it gets worse as we get older because the skin gets drier. It's the build-up of wax that's the issue. This tends to block the ear canal and cause deafness, pain and a sensation of disorientation. Its removal is as liberating as a successful trip to the toilet after three days' constipation!

How do we get rid of it?

The doctor or practice nurse will have a look in your ear with an auroscope – that's the thing with the light on it and a pointed end to see into the ear canal; you won't see anything with the naked eye. If the ear is blocked, soften the wax with a few drops of over-the-counter remedy, or almond oil or olive oil heated to body temperature. Do this two or three times a day for five days and the wax is likely to fall out. If it doesn't, then it's back to the doctor, who might advise syringing.

When I was a little girl, my dad used to syringe the local priest's ears using a big metal syringe and collecting the gunk into a bowl. But times have moved on and there is now a nifty machine so the doctor can squirt water under controlled pressure into the ear to help push the wax out. It's is far more dignified and far safer.

Prone to wax?

People often ask me why they keep getting ear wax. It's normal, but if you use cotton buds you tend to push it in further and the wax gets impacted. The cotton buds also irritate the ear, which in turn causes more wax. If you have a narrow ear canal, you have hairy ears or you are older, you are more likely to have problems too.

Why won't the doctor syringe my ears?

No doctor will syringe your ears unless the wax has been softened first. This is common practice as blindly syringing ears without first softening the wax can risk perforation of the ear drum. If there is any infection, if you have had a perforated ear drum in the last twelve months or if you have previously had difficulty or severe pain with syringing, we might suggest that it isn't a good idea. If it really needs to be done but can't, you might end up seeing an ENT specialist who will vacuum it out with a special suction apparatus.

Worried about wax?

This is one you can't possibly self-diagnose! Ask the doctor or nurse to look in your ears. If there is only a small amount of wax, you are likely to be able to release it just with wax-dissolving drops. Hopi ear candles are another 'home-help' method and use heat to soften the wax; they are also used for other many ear conditions by complementary practitioners. Personally, I would not advise them as a treatment as the result is often that the wax is pushed in further and your hair gets charred. If simple drops don't remove the wax, make it your doctor's problem.

Tips   *Deafness can be a symptom of ear wax. If you are being told you have the TV on too loud, get your ears checked as they could be blocked with wax.*

If you are waxy, use drops periodically as you are less likely to become totally blocked.

Myth   *If you have your ears syringed once, you have to keep having it done. No, you only need it again if you become blocked again.*

EARS THAT ACHE, POP OR BLOCK

Most of us either remember childhood ear infections or have looked after a miserable child with one. In adults though, infection is not always the cause of pain. Tell your doctor how long the pain has been going on and whether there is any deafness, dizziness, nausea, buzzing or popping. You should also mention whether you have recently been flying or diving. In addition, is there any gunk coming out of your ear?

What's the problem?

Ear ache is often due to a build-up of wax, or it could be due to an infection. A perforated ear drum or swimmer's itch after a holiday can also be the culprit. And problems with the tubes between the back of the nose and the middle ear – the eustachian tubes – can have an effect.

Eustachian tube dysfunction

Eustachian tube dysfunction – ETD – is common. The eustachian tube is about 2cm (1in) long and opens when you swallow or yawn to balance the pressure between the outer and inner ear. It can, however, play up and not open, resulting in a pressure build-up outside the ear, stretching and pushing the ear drum inwards. As with an ordinary drum, it will then not function as well in transmitting sound, affecting your hearing. It will also cause pain and popping. The usual cause is a mild infection.

THE MIDDLE EAR

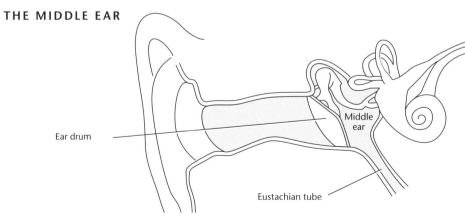

Ear drum

Middle ear

Eustachian tube

Infections

Middle ear infections, i.e. those behind the ear drum, can cause ear ache and the sensation of a blocked ear. They are usually so painful they will have you in tears. They are most common in growing children. Swimmer's ear or otitis externa occurs when the outer ear canal becomes infected after exposure to water in a swimming pool or shower. Those with flaky skin from eczema or psoriasis can be more prone as the mixture of water, skin flakes and bugs provides a healthy reservoir for infection.

Perforation

Beware the cotton bud as overvigorous budding can perforate your ear drum. Flying or diving with an ear infection, trauma such as a head injury or exposure to loud noise, such as a bomb blast, or occasionally a severe infection can cause perforation.

What should I do?

You can't look into your own ear so see your doctor. Middle ear infections are often treated with antibiotics and painkillers. External ear infections can, if mild, be fixed with topical antibiotic drops, sprays or creams. Very severe infection may warrant a clean-out – aural toilet – which basically means the muck gets sucked out by a specialist with a suction machine. Torn ear drums are usually not treated as they fix themselves in about six to eight weeks. It is vital, however, to keep the ear dry to avoid infection. And you shouldn't fly with a perforated ear drum.

My doctor is making me suffer with ETD – surely this isn't fair?

If the problem is mild, the patient just needs to be patient and the condition will disappear in a week or so. In an effort to 'unpop' your ears' you can try to breath out with your nose and mouth blocked – the Valsalva manoeuvre. Steroid nasal sprays, decongestant sprays or antihistamines may help if you have associated hay fever or respiratory symptoms, but antibiotics won't make any difference. If the symptoms go on for four weeks or more, go back to the doctor – you will probably need a further assessment by an ENT doctor.

Tip *If your ears are painful when you're travelling by plane, block your nose and mouth and blow out as if you were inflating a balloon – it helps relieve the pressure.*

TINNITUS

Tinnitus comes from the Latin word for ringing. It refers to buzzing, hissing, pulsating, ringing, whistling or any sort of jingle-jangle in the ear. Oddly, there is nothing on the outside producing this sound, but our brain interprets connections between itself and the nerves in our ears and thinks there is. It's like your mobile phone not actually ringing but making a noise due to interference from the TV or radio. As a population, one in seven of us will experience tinnitus at some point of our lives. For one in two hundred, it can be life-impacting.

What causes it?

Have you ever been to a rock concert and had a buzzing in your ears for several days afterwards? That's tinnitus, and the most common cause is decibel damage. Recurrent exposure to noise, such as shooting, head phones, rock concerts or drilling, can cause noise-induced hearing loss and tinnitus. Other causes include ear wax, low iron levels, fluid in the ears, infection, stress and head injury. Some drugs such as aspirin or antibiotics can cause tinnitus, and problems with the teeth and jaws can also be implicated.

How can a doctor diagnose a noise that only I can hear?

Won't they think I'm daft? No, not at all. We are used to dealing with tinnitus and are adept at distinguishing it from other conditions. Discuss what you mean by tinnitus and how the noise affects you. Mention any deafness and any exposure, past or present, to noise. Tell the doctor about any dizziness or headaches you may be experiencing. If there is a family history of these, it helps the doctor to know. Your doctor will examine your ears, nose and throat. Your blood pressure will be checked, as may your iron levels and your thyroid gland function by means of a blood test.

Will I need to see a specialist?

If the cause is not obvious, yes, you will be referred to an ENT specialist. He or she will examine you, do a formal hearing test and often refer you for a scan of your brain and middle ear to see what's going on inside.

What might the specialist say?

Often no treatable cause is found for tinnitus. Don't be disappointed– it's actually reassuring to know nothing sinister is going on inside. An acoustic neuroma is a tumour on the nerve of hearing and requires prompt surgical action. Menière's disease may also be a cause; this is a problem within the ear canal and is associated with deafness and dizziness.

What's the prognosis?

Tinnitus can be transient, such as after a concert, but beware as it is a sign that your ears have been exposed to very high-level noise. Continue the exposure and you could suffer long-term damage – you'll lose the beat of the music due to deafness but gain the long-term drumming of tinnitus. As we get older, tinnitus can occur in association with deafness, usually above the age of sixty. If a cause can be found for your tinnitus and can be eliminated, for example wax in the ear, this should effect a cure. Often, however, if we can't identify a cause that can be eliminated, you are likely to be stuck with it. As time goes by though you tend to adapt to it. Background noise tends to mask it and is a must during quiet times like bedtime. Beware not to expose yourself to high levels of noise or get a build-up of wax in your ears as this will aggravate it. If you have Menière's disease, you will usually be treated with drugs to stabilise your ear receptor cells. An acoustic neuroma is treated by surgery. If you have persistent life-impacting tinnitus, antidepressants may be prescribed. And if the buzzing really is driving you mad, join a support group – it really helps to talk to other tinnitus sufferers.

DEAFNESS

If you suddenly go deaf overnight, don't despair. The most likely cause is that you have got wax in your ear. Infections and eustachian tube dysfunction, which are dealt with earlier in this chapter, are also common causes. Recent attendance at a very loud rock gig may have also depleted you of decibels. These types of deafness tend to be transient. Deafness that has a slower onset and associated symptoms is, however, unlikely to be resolved by a quick examination at the doctor's.

Conductive deafness

This occurs when the sounds cannot pass freely into the ear – they are interrupted for example by wax, by an infection or by a torn ear drum. Sometimes you can get an abnormal growth of bone in the ear, called otosclerosis, and this also interrupts the conduction of sound waves.

Sensorineural deafness

This occurs when the nerve fibres get damaged so the sound can get in but it cannot be interpreted properly as there is a problem with the transmission. Exposure to loud noise can be a cause, as can some prescription medicines, a head injury, a tumour or a genetic predisposition.

What should I do?

If you are worried that you turn the TV up loudly, constantly say 'Pardon?' or have difficulty hearing in the presence of background noise, talk to your doctor. You may need a hearing test. Nine million people in the UK are affected by deafness.

Tell your doctor about other symptoms such as dizziness or buzzing in your ear, as well as about any noise exposure past or present. Your doctor will look in your ears and is also likely to get a tuning fork out to test whether the problem lies in the capturing of the sounds, the transmission of the sounds or both. The doctor is then likely to refer you for formal testing. Audiometry is carried out in a sound-proofed booth and can both confirm your deafness and locate where the fault lies.

Sounds easy?

A hearing aid can be worn if the sound coming in needs to be amplified. This will, however, not actually cure the underlying problem – it will just help you hear the sound better. If there is a problem with the nerves of hearing, i.e. sensorineural deafness, a cochlear implant may be surgically inserted. This stimulates the nerves of hearing to help create a sound. Remember that deafness is an invisible disability and that it not only causes a physical problem, but also has huge social implications for affected individuals and those around them.

Can I prevent it?

If you engage in noisy activities such as shooting and clubbing, protect your ears. And if you are permanently mooching around to the tunes in your personal MP3 player, remember that prolonged exposure may make you lose the music altogether. If you cannot hear external noise or if the person next to you can hear your music, it's too loud for comfort and safety and you are risking long-term damage to your ears, by which of course I mean deafness.

If you are exposed to 85 decibels of noise or above at work, you are required by law to wear ear protectors, but most concerts and clubs emit about 100 decibels! So although an estimated 70 per cent of the population above seventy years of age have some hearing loss, the gap is closing thanks to the irresponsible use of personal stereos and not plugging our ears at gigs or clubs. If you have been left buzzing for a few days after a good night out, it's a sign that you have already strained your ears with excess sounds.

Rule of thumb

Any sound that you can feel as well as hear is not healthy. Lose the boom or lose your hearing.

Joints

7

Be it an ache or a pain, with 206 bones in our body, there is bound to be something of interest here.

REPETITIVE STRAIN INJURY

We have now coined the phrase WRULD, which stands for work-related upper limb disorder. The term RSI – repetitive strain injury – is somewhat outdated, but most of us still use it. The condition is generally seen in those who work in factories or use a computer, the symptoms stemming from doing the same activity repeatedly or for long periods of time. The problems are generally seen in the forearm, elbow, wrist, fingers and neck.

What causes it?

Various symptoms can arise from repetitive or sustained activity, like, for example tennis elbow or writer's cramp. These activities can give rise to problems such as inflammation of the tendons or pressure on the nerves in the particular area. We define RSI as type 1 if we can give the condition a medical name, and as type 2 if we're not able to define it.

Symptoms

You'll find that you will often get pain and tenderness in the muscles and joints when you are doing the relevant activity. You may also experience pins and needles, numbness and cramp, and you may notice a change in the colour or temperature of the skin. You tend to be at increased risk if your posture is poor, if you do repetitive activities and if you don't take enough breaks.

Treatments If you think you have a work-related upper limb problem, seek help from your doctor as taking early action can prevent long-term problems. If your doctor can diagnose the exact cause, this can be treated appropriately. It is imperative that you also have a work station assessment by a physiotherapist to check out the ergonomics of your desk set-up. We wouldn't sit and watch a film in an uncomfortable chair, yet many of us adopt the posture of a contortionist while carrying out our daily duties.

No answers

If the clue to the diagnosis isn't apparent, you are likely to be referred to a specialist, who may be either an orthopaedic specialist or a rheumatologist. However, there still may not be an answer, and you may be defined as having RSI type 2, in which no specific cause is found. Unfortunately, this is much more difficult to manage.

The law

Your employer has a legal duty to prevent staff developing work-related upper limb disorder, so is obliged to do a risk assessment on your work station and improve it to prevent any deterioration in your condition. RSI is no new entity, and your employer should be familiar with it. As far back as one hundred and sixty years ago, writer's cramp was reported in the British Civil Service with the introduction of the steel pen nib. And a swift rise in RSI disorders was reported in the late 1970s to mid 80s as typewriters were replaced by computer key boards.

RSI at what cost?

Most RSI gets better through simple measures such as desk changes, rest or alternate work practices. However, type 2 RSI tends to go on for longer and can become chronic, with major implications for the workplace and the economy. RSI is a large and growing problem across the whole of Europe, with a staggering two thirds of workers being at risk. In the UK alone, it is estimated that there are half a million sufferers. A prompt recognition of the problem pays dividends and will decrease your sickness absence.

SPRAINED ANKLE

I felt that this had to be included in a women's health bible as so many of us come to grief in our stilettos. Indeed, six out of every thousand of us seek medical advice related to this subject each year.

Type of trauma

Your ankle can be injured by twisting in two main directions. Your feet can turn inwards, which is known as an inversion injury and tends to occur in 90 per cent of cases. This results in the pain occurring on the outer aspect of the ankle. Turning outwards is known as an eversion injury and is the less common variety; it is generally the result of a twisting movement. Here the pain occurs on the inner aspect of the ankle. You will often feel the sensation of something giving way, and you may feel a snap. Essentially, what is happening is that you are stretching or tearing the elastic ligaments supporting the ankle joint.

Symptoms

There will generally be pain, swelling and bruising.

Treatment   It really is important to rest for the first forty-eight hours. Elevate the ankle, preferably to a level higher than your heart. This necessitates propping it up on books when you are in bed! Ice it with a pack of frozen peas for twenty minutes every four hours. And compress the swelling by means of a support bandage worn by day but removed at night.

Rehabilitation   If at all possible, try to get physiotherapy for a badly sprained ankle as it will heal more quickly. Stay off sport for six weeks with a bad sprain, and even with a minor sprain stay out of your stilettos for a couple of weeks.

When do I need an X-ray?

If you cannot weight bear, the ankle is very painful and swollen or the symptoms are worsening rather than improving, seek medical advice.

BACK PAIN

Ask an orthopaedic surgeon why we get back pain and their retort is usually that we were bred to walk on four limbs and not two. But with 80 per cent of the population suffering from back pain at some point in their lives, it's not very helpful to suggest the solution is to walk on all fours! Back pain is the second most common reason – after the common cold – for missed work days in those under forty-five.

Back anatomy basics

The bones of the spine are interconnected and called vertebrae; we have twenty-four in total. They are separated by discs that act as shock absorbers, allowing the spine the flexibility to bend. The spinal cord leads off the base of the brain and runs though the spine in the neck and chest area. It does not run through the lower back (the lumbar

THE ANATOMY OF THE SPINE

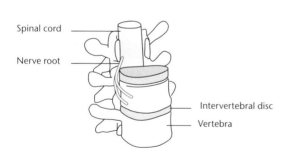

Spinal cord

Nerve root

Intervertebral disc

Vertebra

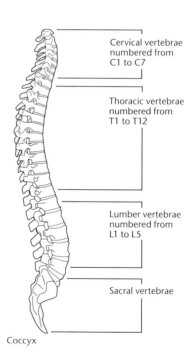

Cervical vertebrae numbered from C1 to C7

Thoracic vertebrae numbered from T1 to T12

Lumber vertebrae numbered from L1 to L5

Sacral vertebrae

Coccyx

spine), but instead the nerves for the lower end of the back come off the end of the spinal cord like a horse's tail.

What is the cause of back pain?

Patients often find it frustrating to be told that in almost 95 per cent of cases we cannot fully identify a cause; we dress this up by calling it musculoskeletal. Five per cent of cases are caused by pressure on or irritation of a nerve coming out of the spinal cord. This may be caused by muscle spasm following an injury, a jolt or a sprain to the spine. It can also be due to a problem with a slipped disc. Pain is felt along the course of the sciatic nerve, so it can go from the buttock to the back of the leg and into the foot. We call this type of pain sciatica.

Non-specific back pain

As the name suggests, this isn't due to anything specific, although it doesn't mean that your doctor can't work out the cause. It may be due to a strained muscle, a ligament, minor problems with a disc or a problem with a facet joint, i.e. one of the joints between the vertebrae. It often comes on after lifting but sometimes just arrives without warning or incident.

What are the risk factors?

Being middle aged, having a family history of back pain, pregnancy, stress, prolonged sitting, excess weight and poor posture.

What are the sinister signs?

- Pain that quickly worsens for no apparent reason
- Pain that is constant irrespective of rest
- Pain that occurs while in bed
- Numbness accompanying the pain
- Weakness accompanying the pain
- Early morning stiffness
- Associated incontinence
- Numbness around the anus.

What tests should I ask for?

You often won't need any tests to identify the cause for your back pain as it will be non-specific – so X-rays, scans and blood tests won't add to the picture. Fewer than 15 per cent of problems will be diagnosed on X-rays, MRI scans or bone scans, hence why we don't immediately refer you to a radiologist.

What's a slipped disc?

Your discs are jelly-like structures that sit between the vertebrae and absorb shock. These discs can wear out and sometimes bulge or break, resulting in pressure being put on the adjacent nerves. When this happens, there may be sudden severe pain in the back, buttock and down your leg, i.e. sciatica. It can also cause numbness and pins and needles. This generally takes longer to settle down, maybe six weeks.

Progress

Fifty per cent of people will feel relief from back pain in two weeks, and 90 per cent in six weeks. For non-specific back pain, remain active and take pain relief. Lots of people worry about taking painkillers for fear of masking an underlying problem. My advice is to take regular pain relief for the first forty-eight hours. Following on from this, take it before exercise or activities that seem to make the pain worse. Don't wait for the pain to get bad to reach for a painkiller – this just slows your recovery. Your doctor can give you stronger painkillers or a combination of painkillers and muscle relaxants if needed.

A visit to the physiotherapist, chiropractor or osteopath may also help if you are not getting on top of things. They can provide exercises or back manipulation where appropriate. They often use treatments like TENS machines or acupuncture to complement their treatments. Two elements are vital in your progress: try to return to work as soon as possible, and don't take to your bed.

What if there's no improvement

Ongoing back pain despite sensible management warrants further referral. Epidural injections (similar to those given in labour) may be an option for back pain and inflammation around the spinal nerves, for example sciatica. Spinal surgery is only required in under 1 per cent of patients. Many hospitals run back rehabilitation programmes that can be very helpful for chronic sufferers. The aim is to get you to lead as normal a life as possible rather than having your back rule your life.

Why have I been given antidepressants for my back?

Amitriptyline in low doses is often given at night for back pain. It helps with sleep and seems to block pain impulses, so is often helpful in chronic pain. It is a known fact that people with long-term back problems can become depressed, so watch for signs of this as it will impede your recovery.

Tips

Beware back pain as it may be a symptom of a foot, knee or hip problem.

Pilates helps to strengthen your core muscles and is excellent for those who sit at a desk all day.

Myth

Bed rest is best for back pain. No, it isn't. Unless your doctor advises you otherwise, you are best to remain active, but not 'gym active', to prevent your muscles from going into spasm and your joints getting stiff.

CARPAL TUNNEL SYNDROME

Despite sounding like some form of claustrophobia, this actually involves your hand. Never heard of it? Well there is a one in twenty chance it will strike you in your lifetime. It tends to occur from the mid-forties right into the sixties but can happen at any time and is common in pregnancy.

What are the symptoms?

Your hand and fingers feel painful and burn, and there may be a feeling of pins and needles, numbness or that sensation as if you have slept on your arm. The pain tends to be worst at night and is relieved by hanging the arm over the side of the bed. It's usually the thumb, index finger and middle finger that are affected, plus the half of the ring finger adjacent to these.

So what's the problem down the carpal tunnel?

This tunnel runs from the wrist downwards to the fingers, carrying the tendons that move the fingers. There is also a nerve in there, the median nerve – that's the one that pings if you bang your elbow. For some reason everything seems to get squashed in carpal tunnel syndrome due to a lack of room. Because of this, pressure is put on the nerve and that's why you get symptoms.

CARPAL TUNNEL SYNDROME

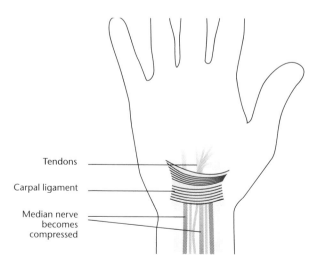

Tendons

Carpal ligament

Median nerve becomes compressed

How does it happen in the first place?

We don't really know, but it tends to cluster in families. One in four people with it have relatives similarly affected. It is more common in people with joint problems such as gout or rheumatoid arthritis. It also tends to be more prevalent in those who are carrying too much weight or tend to retain fluid – this is probably why it happens in pregnancy. It can also happen after you have broken your wrist or if you have thyroid gland problems.

How does the doctor diagnose it?

Your symptoms are often the key. The doctor can confirm the diagnosis by getting you to hold your wrist in a specific way that brings on the symptoms. If the diagnosis isn't definite, there's a further test called a nerve conduction study. This basically tests the nerve's electrical signals and shows they aren't sparking efficiently because they are being compressed in the tunnel.

What next?

First, see a physiotherapist. They can fit you with a splint. Anti-inflammatory tablets may also be of benefit as they kill pain and decrease the swelling in the carpal tunnel. Steroid tablets can be resorted to for two to four weeks if the condition is very severe; alternatively, a steroid injection can be given into the wrist. This is, however, not a long-term solution as the recurrent use of steroids is not safe.

Surgery

This is called carpal tunnel release surgery; in it, the surgeon makes a cut in the carpal ligament to make more space in the tunnel. It's usually a day case procedure and you won't normally have a general anaesthetic, although the area that's being operated on will of course be given a local anaesthetic. The procedure can be carried out by a specialist orthopaedic or plastic surgeon, and it will be about six weeks before you are fully functioning again.

Self-help

It goes without saying that if you are overweight, try and shed some of the extra kilos – it can not only help with the carpal tunnel syndrome, but also be of benefit if you end up needing an operation. Avoid doing repetitive movements, such as vacuuming or painting, that will aggravate the problem. I'm not saying go on a total housework strike, but if you need to do repetitive movements, take rest periods and do simple stretching exercises such as squeezing a softball.

FROZEN SHOULDER

When this happens, the shoulder literally freezes, and movement is painful and reduced. The shoulder behaves a bit like a hinge that hasn't been oiled and, boy, is it both sore and also debilitating. Doctors call this condition adhesive capsulitis.

How would I know if my shoulder was frozen – would it be cold?

No, the freezing part has nothing to do with temperature, but more indicates stiffness. Your shoulder becomes very painful and stiff. Any movement or any pressure, for example even sleeping on it, will cause pain. If you try and flap your arms like a bird, you won't be able to because of the pain and stiffness. Rotating your shoulder to do up your bra may also be impossible or incredibly painful.

Who gets this?

One in fifty adults get this at some point in their lives, but if you have diabetes and you are between forty and sixty, you are more likely to do so. And guess what girls? – we

ANATOMY OF THE SHOULDER

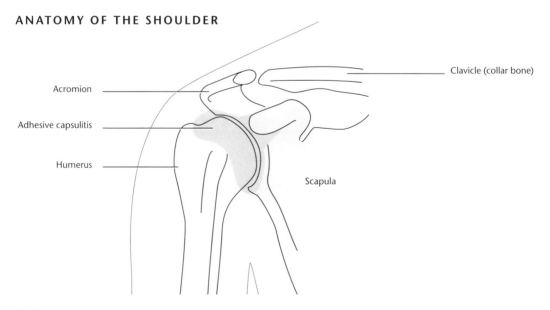

Clavicle (collar bone)

Acromion

Adhesive capsulitis

Humerus

Scapula

get it more often than the boys do. Those who suffer from Parkinson's disease, thyroid problems or heart disease are also more likely to develop it.

If you write with your right hand, you are likely to get it in your left shoulder and vice versa. Just to frustrate you even further, 20 per cent of people who get it on one side tend to get it on the other side at some point.

What causes it?

Like lots of medical problems, we really don't know for sure. It can sometimes come on after even a minor injury to the shoulder, such as walking into a door, or after a more significant trauma such as a fall. But, irritatingly, there is often no history of trauma whatsoever.

How do you diagnose it?

The doctor will often diagnose it by listening to your symptoms and doing an examination. An X-ray is not done as this is likely to be normal. Sometimes, if your symptoms are complex, you will be referred for an MRI (magnetic resonance imaging) scan as this can show up lots more than X-rays, for example tendons and muscles.

How does it progress?

The 'freezing' part occurs first, with the joint becoming painful and gradually becoming stiff with limited movement. This can last for between two and nine months.

Next it reaches the 'frozen' phase where pain becomes less and the stiffness worsens, so any movement becomes very restricted. Typically, the person cannot raise their arm above their head. This is because the shoulder joint is a ball and socket joint.

Think back to your childhood dolls to understand this. Your upper arm is the ball, and it sits inside the socket of the shoulder blade. An elastic (stretchy) capsule surrounds the shoulder joint and is maximally stretched when you raise your arm above your head – hence this is the most difficult movement to perform in frozen shoulder because the elasticity has been lost. So fixing the mirror inside your car to do your lipstick is a nightmare. This stage can go on for three months to up to a full year.

Finally, the shoulder decides to thaw, and the symptoms gradually lessen and movement improves. But this could take six months or even two full years.

How do you help defrost this frozen shoulder?

▌ Act quickly! If you think your shoulder might be seizing up, seek help as soon as you can. Anti-inflammatory painkillers help the inflammation in the joint and also kill the pain – you can use over-the-counter ibuprofen or a doctor's prescription for diclofenac, for example. However, these don't suit everyone – for example, those with asthma or a stomach ulcer – so check first.

▌ Exercises are very helpful as they prevent further stiffening. Ideally, therefore, you should see a physiotherapist.

▌ Steroid injections can be given to help decrease the pain and inflammation, but these don't always work and they can't be given too frequently because of their side-effects.

▌ Surgery is a last resort but can be done to release the capsule, i.e. the cover, of the shoulder joint and restore movement. Again, it isn't always successful.

▌ Having a frozen shoulder is frustrating. It limits us in our daily activities, so act quickly to prevent it becoming a menace for months and months.

FROZEN SHOULDER REHABILITATION EXCERCISES

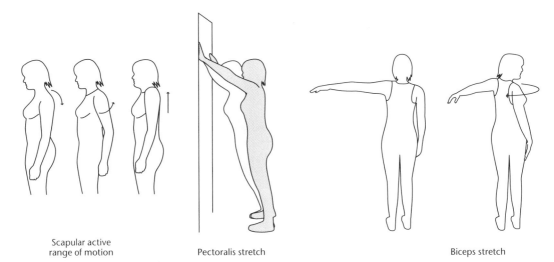

Scapular active
range of motion

Pectoralis stretch

Biceps stretch

BUNIONS

Nine out of ten people who get bunions are ladies. Have a look at your feet; is your big toe angled in towards your second toe? This is the deformity, and the bunion is the consequence of the deformity. We doctors call it hallux valgus, and it's essentially a bump on the side of your big toe.

What causes bunions?

Before you go throwing out your Jimmy Choos – although footwear has been implicated – there is also evidence that women's ligaments are more lax and that this predisposes us to bunions. But it makes sense that squeezing our toes into our fashion numbers is going to crowd them and not make life easy for the big toe. Although we see bunions in populations who do not wear shoes, such as Amazonian tribes, it is rare. It is also true that you are more likely to get bunions if your parents or grandparents suffered, so check the family tree and choose your footwear accordingly.

A BUNION

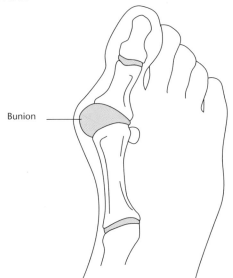

Bunion

What's the big problem with them?

Aesthetically, bunions aren't pretty! More importantly, your bunion can become inflamed, and a collection of fluid can form around it and cause pain. It will then be red and tender to touch. The big toe can also push the other toes as it leans inwards, making walking difficult. And because of overcrowding, you are more likely to get corns and calluses. So we are not only talking ugly feet here, we are talking painful feet.

What do you do if you have a bunion?

If you've got a bunion, choose wide-fitting shoes. Avoid slip-ons as they need to be tighter to stay on; much better to go for laces or straps instead. High heels put your toes under pressure as all your weight gets transferred onto the balls of your feet, so opt for wedges.

If you are having problems, see a podiatrist. These are people who are trained in all matters to do with feet, from fallen arches to nasty nails. A podiatrist will watch you walking and do a biomechanical assessment. They can assess your gait, see if there are any mechanical problems with how you walk and correct them with an orthotic. This is a bespoke insert for your shoe, tailor-made for your foot by taking a plaster of Paris cast impression of it.

Wearing orthotics will ease the pressure on the bunions and as such prevent pain and deterioration. You can also be fitted with night splints, which keep the toes straight at night and help realignment.

Tips *If you have a flare-up of bunion pain after a night of dancing in high heels, get a bag of frozen peas on the bunion for twenty minutes every two hours and take an anti-inflammatory. This will kill the pain and help with the inflammation.*

If your toes are starting to look bendy, try toe aerobics. With your feet together, bring your toes together to meet in the middle. Do this six to eight times a day.

If your bunions are worsening

See a foot and ankle surgeon, who can cut the bunion out. There are over a hundred different operations, so just because your neighbour had one procedure, that doesn't mean it's the one to suit you. Remember that this is the last resort after conservative measures as if you opt for an op, you will be off your feet for four weeks.

Like Cinderella, make sure the shoe fits. There needs to be 1cm (half an inch) between your big toe and the front of your shoe. And throw out any shoes, however pretty, that 'murder' your feet.

GOUT

Do girls get gout? Oh yes, and as well as not being glamorous, it's unbelievably painful. About one in a hundred people are susceptible to it, although mostly men.

What happens?
Gout occurs because a product of metabolism called uric acid usually lost in the urine builds up in the blood and crystallises in the joints. Classically, gout strikes at night, and on wakening you have an inflamed, shiny, swollen, red, hot, painful big toe. This is the most common site but any joint can be affected.

But as I'm a woman, I'm not that likely to get it, right?
Wrong, we see it in women after the menopause, who take water tablets for swollen ankles or high blood pressure, or are obese. Gout has been recorded for over two thousand years and has always been associated with excess, for example of beer, wine, port, oysters, mussels, anchovies or sardines, all of which increase uric acid. Lentils, asparagus and spinach can also cause problems, as can dehydration.

Is it that bad?
Yes, because it's awfully painful – and because repeated attacks damage the joint and leave you with persistent pain. It's easy to diagnose, but a blood test may be sent off to check the uric acid. An attack will last about two weeks and requires prescription medication to abate it. Strong anti-inflammatories like indometacin (indomethacin), diclofenac or naproxen are usually given. These aren't suitable if you have a stomach ulcer or asthma. Colchicine is an alternative, but it can give horrid diarrhoea too. If you get more than two attacks of gout a year, you will require regular allopurinol. High uric acid also makes you prone to kidney stones, another terribly painful problem.

I'm nowhere near the menopause, so am I safe?
Binge drinking, high-protein 'Atkins-type' diets, sugary drinks, Marmite munching and excess weight all put you at risk of getting gout whatever your age or sex. It also runs in families so check your family tree.

OSTEOPOROSIS

Our bones are made of a hard outer shell and an inner honeycomb mesh, a bit like a Crunchie bar, if you've had one of those. When the inner honeycomb network becomes less dense, i.e. more holes develop in the 'honeycomb' of the bone, we call this osteoporosis. Despite the fact that you probably stopped growing at sixteen, your bones have remained active and are indeed always in a state of flux.

Who is at risk?

Everyone is at risk. In fact, one in five women over the age of sixty are likely to develop osteoporosis. But beware – it is not simply an older woman's disease. Today's size zero culture is producing a lot of women with a small body frame, and this in itself is a risk factor for osteoporosis. The bigger your body frame, the better – without any excess fat of course. Family history is also a risk factor, so check out old photos of your grandmother to see if she got shorter as she got older as this is often a sign of

DEVELOPMENT OF OSTEOPOROSIS

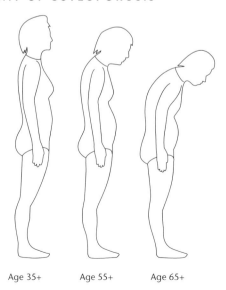

Age 35+   Age 55+   Age 65+

osteoporosis. Keeping within your alcohol units is important as there is good evidence to show that if you deviate and drink outside your fourteen units per week, you are more likely to develop it. Smoking is also bad news for bones.

What about diet and exercise?

What's in your diet is really important, and faddy diets devoid of calcium, such as high-protein diets or dairy-free diets, may cause issues with bone mass. Lack of exercise is another contributing factor as we need regular weightbearing exercise to keep our bones healthy. Conversely, excessive exercise that interferes with periods, i.e. causes them to be irregular or absent, increases your risk of osteoporosis. Extreme dieting and anorexia are also implicated.

Do other illnesses make me more likely to have porous bones?

Yes, I'm afraid so. An overactive thyroid gland or diabetes can thin the bones. So too can problems with your adrenal glands (which are situated just over your kidneys and control your natural level of steroids) or your pituitary gland (which is situated in your brain and controls your hormones). Menopause is probably best known for making bones more porous. Diseases such as coeliac disease or Crohn's disease that affect your gut can have an impact on your stores of calcium. Patients who take regular steroid medication – those who have arthritis, for example – are more at risk. This should not be confused with taking steroids via an inhaler for asthma or in creams for eczema, as the risk with these is negligible.

My joints would ache if I had it, wouldn't they?

Not necessarily. The first time that osteoporosis gets diagnosed tends, ironically, to be when you break a bone, i.e. when its too late. The lifetime risk of a hip fracture in a woman aged fifty is greater than that of breast cancer or heart disease as it is estimated to be one in six. The scary thing is that 50 per cent of women may be permanently limited in activities such as climbing stairs or shopping after this. Ladies often slip on the pavement or end up breaking a rib while coughing, and this is the first clue to the brittle status of their bones. It has aptly been called the silent epidemic.

Are there any visual clues?

Getting shorter is a clue as you tend to lose height in osteoporosis. You may also develop a hump in your back called a dowager's hump, a bit like a buffalo hump. You adopt a stooping posture. If you frequently suffer from broken bones, you should raise questions of why your bones are breaking. The most common ones to snap in osteoporosis are the hip, wrist and spine. Another clue may be on your plate – if your diet is devoid of calcium, for example in cheese, yoghurt and milk, you may be heading for trouble. Believe it or not, cereals are a great source of calcium, so it's not just dairy, dairy, dairy.

How do you diagnose it?

Osteoporosis is often picked up on a plain X-ray done for another reason, such as a chest X-ray. The gold standard for diagnosing it is the bone density scan, which we call a DEXA scan. Cutting through the scientific jargon, this is a special scanner that uses X-rays that can grade how dense your bones are. There is no blood test available for osteoporosis, and although the level of calcium can be measured in the blood, it will neither confirm nor deny your bone density status.

Are there porosis-preventing pills?

Yes, and they have been shown to decrease the risk of fractures by at least 50 per cent. To understand how they work, you need to get a glimpse of how the bone mechanics work. The building block of bone is calcium, but for this to be available and active you need vitamin D3. This is made in the body when sunlight shines on the skin and can also be taken in via food and supplements. Bone mass starts to decline at about age thirty-five, and the reabsorption of bone then overtakes its re-formation.

Bisphosphonates

These drugs work by replacing lost bone and preventing further loss. Think of the bisphosphonates as the builders who come in to replace your roof tiles and strengthen the roof to prevent further loss. They are the mainstay of treatment. The problem, however, is that they do not easily get from the gut into the body, so they need to be taken on an empty stomach, sitting up and with lots of water. These restrictions make them a nuisance to take either at night or first thing in the morning. The good news, however, is that the bisphosphonates alendronate and risedronate need to be taken only once a week, and ibandronate only once a month. They can, however, cause side-effects of gut irritation and stomach ulcers.

In addition, you will be prescribed a combination of calcium and vitamin D. Many women hate taking these as they taste chalky and may make you belch or pass wind, but they're a must if the bisphosphonate medication is to work. Diet and sunshine alone won't suffice.

Other drugs

HRT is also used for the treatment of osteoporosis in suitable patients. Strontium ranelate, raloxifene or parathyroid hormone peptides are also used, but the most likely prescription you will emerge with is for our friend the bisphosphonate and a calcium–vitamin D combo.

Progress

Your treatment will be lifelong. Stop it and the disease progresses, with all the serious side-effects of fractures. Remember too that regular weightbearing exercise and diet and lifestyle modifications are applicable as well – you don't escape the recommendation for thirty minutes weightbearing exercise five times a week. It's all beneficial.

Prevention is better than cure

Lifestyle issues of exercise, diet, cigarettes and alcohol play a huge role here. Start boosting your calcium now by drinking a pint of milk a day, and your vitamin D3 by eating tuna and sardines. Remember that your bone density is at its maximum in your twenties and starts going downhill in your thirties, so take action early.

Tips   *Beware the BMI of 19 or under (see page 255) as it puts you at risk of osteoporosis.*

      A pint of semi-skimmed milk contains more calcium than a pint of full-fat milk.

Myth   *Men don't suffer from osteoporosis. Of course they do!*

Mental health

8

The brain is the most powerful organ in the body. Discover how to know your own mind and when to ask for help.

DEPRESSION

Depression is characterised by low mood and a loss of interest or pleasure in activities. It's not just a frame of mind – it's a serious medical condition – and 15 per cent of people have a bout of depression at some point. It's twice as common in women as men. The person generally feels worthless, tired and sad, with a loss of appetite and problems sleeping or concentrating. They can also be preoccupied by morbid thoughts. Libido tends to be low, and sexual and interpersonal relationships suffer due to moodiness and irritability.

What increases your risks of depression?

Doctors refer to 'life events', so a death, a separation or a financial burden may serve as a trigger. Drugs such as cannabis and excessive alcohol are also implicated, as are chronic medical problems such as back pain, psoriasis or heart disease. In addition, there may be a family history of depression.

Tests There aren't really any tests for depression, but blood tests can rule out other problems, especially with physical symptoms such as tiredness that can have other causes too. Iron deficiency, lack of vitamin B12, thyroid problems and the menopause may cause similar symptoms. So too can hormonal treatments such as the oral contraceptive pill, epilepsy, Alzheimer's disease, cancer and withdrawal from cigarettes or alcohol.

Treatments Recognition that there is a problem is often the first step. Issues related to past events such as death or abuse need to be managed through counselling and cognitive-behavioural therapy (CBT). This works on how we think related to how we feel, and tries to change our thought patterns. Symptoms frequently improve with talking therapy, and medication may never be needed. Family or couple therapy is used if there are issues relating to others. Psychotherapy works on our childhood experiences and relates them to how we feel now.

Tablets do, however, have a place, and it's always difficult when a patient refuses point blank to go down the medical route when presenting with severe depression.

There is often a preconceived notion that resorting to medication is in some way giving in. But it's the opposite and successful medication allows you to 'get on with it'.

Understanding brain chemistry helps to understand the rationale behind taking medication. Serotonin and noradrenaline (norepinephrine) are neurotransmitters – chemicals that act to transmit messages between nerve cells. When they are released from nerve cells, they are found to lift our mood. But if they are stuck to nerve cells, this effect goes. Imagine noradrenaline and serotonin as mobile phone networks – if they are blocked, the happy message isn't getting through, but unblocking them with chemicals lets the happy message get through as their circulating levels rise. SSRIs (selective serotonin reuptake inhibitors) are used most frequently in the UK, America and Australia and are by and large safe and well tolerated. They block the serotonin receptors, so serotonin doesn't get bound up on them. Examples include citalopram, paroxetine and our well-publicised friend fluoxetine (Prozac).

The SNRI (serotonin–noradrenaline reuptake inhibitors) group are another family of drugs that affect serotonin and noradrenaline. Examples of these are venlafaxine and duloxetine. These are often used as first-line medications in the USA and other countries, but in the UK tend to be used for more severe depression and when SSRIs have proved ineffectual. The NASSA (noradrenaline and specific serotonergic antidepressant) group, for example mirtazapine, of antidepressants work on noradrenaline and specific serotonin receptors.

Tricyclic antidepressants and monoamine oxidase inhibitors are older antidepressants. I have rarely prescribed the latter as newer drugs are better, but they are still very much in use in the UK. They too work on the levels of these brain neurotransmitters, but they tend to have more generalised side-effects outside the brain than newer drugs do. The one most commonly used is amitriptyline.

Problems with pills If you and your doctor together decide that medication is right for you, there are a few features you should be aware of. Your symptoms may become much worse in the first few days after you start the tablets. The other key thing is that they won't work immediately – they often take two to four weeks to kick in. Side-effects include nausea, dizziness, headache, changes in appetite and libido, and fatigue. Not everybody gets every side-effect listed inside the box – most people don't get any at all. And as time goes on, the side-effects become less noticeable. Over 50 per cent of patients feel better on antidepressants. The older tricyclic antidepressants (e.g. amitriptyline) can cause a dry mouth, blurred vision, drowsiness and problems passing urine, but these tend to lessen with time.

Will I become addicted to antidepressants? No, they don't have an addictive profile. However, stopping them abruptly can give withdrawal symptoms such as dizziness, nausea and feelings of flu or electric shock. When you and your doctor come to the decision that it's time to come off the tablets, it's best to taper the dose down over a few weeks to limit side-effects. The ideal time to make this decision is when you feel at your best and the depressive cloud has lifted.

Top tips on tablet taking Persevere – most people stop too early as they don't see any benefit. You need to take the tablets every day and not just when you feel down. And check in with your doctor every few weeks. Most patients who leave with no follow-up arranged fail to get better. Talk to the doctor about upping the dosage if it doesn't seem adequate, or changing the medicine if it doesn't seem effective.

Try to avoid drinking alcohol with antidepressants as it can make you feel more depressed, make side-effects worse and make you more intoxicated more quickly. Whatever you do, don't go off your antidepressants so you can drink over the festive season or a holiday. You will undoubtedly suffer a double relapse!

Further care

Depression is usually treated by the family doctor but sometimes, if it's very severe or there's a risk of suicide, a psychiatrist's help may be necessary. This is usually on an outpatient basis but you may need a stay in hospital.

Postnatal depression

One in ten women suffer a bout of depression after giving birth. This generally kicks in a month after birth but can occur any time up to six months. You feel depressed, guilty, anxious, irritable and unable to cope, tired but can't sleep. You may even go off your partner, and your libido drops to zero. A mild version of this is called the baby blues and hits most mothers around day three or four after birth. It is important to seek help for postnatal depression as many women suffer for months if not years. Often little more than increased support and some counselling are needed, but antidepressants are occasionally prescribed.

Seasonal affective disorder

This is a type of winter depression that hits an estimated one in fifty people in the UK, with women twice as likely to suffer as men. The winter months are the worst, and the condition often coincides with changing the clocks. It can last anything from one to five months. General feelings of low mood and negative thoughts are accompanied by a tendency to oversleep, crave carbohydrates and experience poor concentration, a loss of desire to socialise and difficulty in coping with normal activities. It strikes between the ages of eighteen and thirty and is more likely the further you live from the equator. It is thought to be due to an imbalance between your levels of serotonin (happy hormone) and melatonin (jet lag hormone).

Treatment Common sense says that if it is due to a lack of light, light should improve the symptoms. You can purchase a light box that emits at ten times the brightness and intensity of an ordinary bulb. You may need to spend between thirty minutes and two hours exposed to it, but as you are advised to sit nearly a metre (three feet) away from it and not look at it directly, you can get on with your daily activities at the same time. Its effect can be seen within a week, and if nothing happens by six weeks, you are probably one of the unlucky 33 per cent of affected individuals who won't get any benefit. An alternative is to take antidepressants such as SSRIs during the winter months.

Manic depression

This is also called bipolar affective disorder and the sufferer gets extreme swings of mood. This can range from morbid depression with suicidal thoughts and social isolation to manic behaviour where the person dresses flamboyantly, spends excessively, is sexually promiscuous and talks and acts frenetically. Interestingly, about

1 per cent of the population are said to suffer. Men equal women in the bipolar stakes, and one in ten sufferers have an affected relative. Lithium is generally the mainstay of treatment, and patients in the initial stages are managed largely by psychiatry clinics. Treatment is generally long term.

Do people still use shock treatment?

Yes electric shock treatment – electroconvulsive therapy or ECT – is still used by psychiatrists to treat severe depression or prolonged episodes of mania when other treatment has failed. When it was first introduced in the 1930s, there weren't many pharmacological treatments available, so it served its purpose at the time. Its current use is governed by strict guidelines, and it will probably be phased out in time.

Tips   ▌ *Depression can be the first sign of an underlying medical disorder, for example an underactive thyroid gland.*

▌ *Loss of libido may be a clue that you are depressed.*

Myths   ▌ *Stop smoking cannabis and the symptoms will simply disappear. No – it's often a case of too little too late. And the younger you are when you start using cannabis, the greater your risk of developing mental health problems.*

▌ *Antidepressants are addictive. No they're not, so don't worry about taking them.*

INSOMNIA

Insomnia – difficulty initiating and/or maintaining sleep – is the most common sleep complaint in adults: one in ten of us have a long-term problem. Women are affected twice as often as men, but there's no sex difference before puberty.

What causes the problem?

Causes are multiple. Often it's hormonal fluxes, for example during menopause. Any condition that results in chronic pain can cause it, as can restless legs syndrome and bladder problems. Alcohol, cigarettes, caffeine and late-night eating have been implicated. Depression, anxiety and work or domestic factors such as babies or shift work are involved too.

The specifics

Early morning wakening, i.e. wakening at 4am and being unable to get back to sleep, is a classic symptom of depression. Initial insomnia and broken sleep can be a sign of anxiety and stress. Inability to go to sleep at all may signify a period of mania, as in bipolar affective disorder. Those who go on recreational cocaine and alcohol binges will find it hard to 'come down' and often report sleep problems.

Help for insomnia

It goes without saying that a healthy diet, exercise and moderation in alcohol are a must. Avoid eating large amounts late at night or eating spicy foods. Ditch the caffeine culprits such as tea, cola and chocolate before bedtime as they are stimulating. Being overweight affects sleep, so address this too. Use bed only for sleep and not for eating, or TV. Make sure the temperature and noise levels are optimum, and hide the bedroom clock, or you'll watch it tick-tock through the night. If you can't sleep after thirty minutes, get up and do something else, preferably relaxing and in not too bright a light. It's vital to stick to a timetable, even at weekends, and don't cat nap!

Therapy

Cognitive-behavioural therapy can help by changing negative thoughts about sleep, and relaxation therapy is beneficial. The role of acupuncture and hypnosis has not yet been fully verified.

Pills

Doctors are very cautious about prescribing sleeping pills because of the side-effects. Benzodiazepines (diazepam, temazepam) are rarely prescribed for insomnia due to their addictive profile and their impact on performance such as driving the following day. These are reserved for severe intractable cases. The 'Z' medicines (zolpidem and zaleplon) act in a similar fashion but without the side-effects. They should be used for two to five days for transient and not more than four weeks for short-term insomnia.

What about melatonin?

This is the naturally occurring hormone that regulates the sleep pattern and is also the jet lag hormone. It can regulate short-term insomnia and is available to the over-fifty-fives on prescription in the UK. In the USA, it can be bought over the counter, and in Australia you can get it over the counter or on prescription. However, over-the-counter brands may not be fully therapeutic, so talk to your doctor.

Isn't restless legs syndrome all in the mind and not in the limbs?

Wrong! This desire to move the legs when they are at rest is common and often a reason for insomnia. It can feel like the legs are jumping, crampy, numb and downright restless. Oddly enough, this only becomes obvious when the person is lying down trying to relax. Fifty per cent of people have an affected family member. It's more common in women and tends to hit from middle age. The condition is sadly lifelong but can be improved by cutting down on caffeine and alcohol. Checks on iron, vitamin B12 and folic acid and for diabetes are also important. If it's driving you mad, muscle relaxants, drugs used to treat Parkinson's disease or some medications for epilepsy may help. There's no specific medication, so unfortunately it's a case of trial and error.

What about warm milk?

Foods like milk that contain tryptophan are sleep-inducing. Other sources are bananas, honey and poultry, which may explain why we snooze after Sunday lunch.

BODY IMAGE DISORDERS

You are both what you eat and what you don't eat!

Food fuels many emotions. We deny ourselves food as punishment if, for example, we want to lose weight, we overeat protein and carbohydrates if we want to bulk up, we gorge on chocolate because Mr Right has yet again turned out to be Mr Wrong. Food is used as a tool in many emotions; it can be a treat or a torture.

Not happy with how you look?

Many women would like to change some part of their appearance. I for one would like a better set of feet – my own are horrific. Body dysmorphic disorder is a psychiatric condition in which you become preoccupied with a minute bodily flaw such as a freckle, or you imagine there to be defect that is not apparent to others. Classically, it's seen in those who have anorexia – they imagine they are overweight when they are in fact waif-like.

It's difficult to get an accurate estimate of how many women suffer from this disorder; some statistics would say 0.5 to 1 per cent of the female population. This is not a new disorder that has sprung from the size zero culture; it was first identified in 1886 and given its name from the Greek word for misshapen.

But surely it's normal for a woman not to think she looks perfect?

Of course it is! But sufferers of body dysmorphic disorder believe that they are ugly or disgusting, and it is impossible to persuade them otherwise. They are not vain, but they do spend hours looking in the mirror, self-grooming, comparing themselves with models in magazines and obsessing with diet and exercise. They will often seek the help of plastic surgeons and dermatologists to improve their perceived hideous looks. A woman who is suffering from body dysmorphic disorder will spend over an hour a day ruminating about her 'flaw', will feel others tell her she looks fine just because they are being nice and will feel generally ashamed about what she deems to be her ugly appearance. This phenomenon takes over the person's life and inhibits both professional and personal activities.

How common is anorexia?

One in one hundred girls aged between sixteen and eighteen suffer. Forty per cent of those with anorexia make a full recovery, but 30 per cent suffer a long-term problem and the remaining 30 per cent keep their condition under control. So although this is seen as a disorder of the teens and twenties, the problem progresses throughout life. The issue in anorexia is a morbid fear of being fat and an obsession with weight.

Anorexics are classically 15 per cent below the expected weight for their height. They have an element of body dysmorphobia in that they still feel that they are ugly and overweight despite falling into the underweight category. They strictly control their calorie intake, often resorting to strenuous exercise to burn off excess calories. They may also use laxatives and diuretics to achieve the same end.

Why does it occur?

It sometimes starts because you are overweight and have received negative comments. So you begin to diet, and the obsessive dieting gradually descends into anorexia. Low self-esteem and depression are triggers too. It is also more common in perfectionists, ballet dancers, high achievers both academically and in sport, and models. Puberty, peer pressure and family difficulties may serve as triggers.

But surely it's only a phase?

Fifteen per cent of anorexics will die within twenty years if the disorder remains untreated. This is no 'phase' they are going through. The condition can result in problems with the bones, for example osteoporosis, cause periods to stop and interfere with fertility and libido. It affects energy levels, concentration and mood, and often comes with an associated depression and a potential increased risk of suicide. The kidneys and liver suffer, as does general health because of a lack of nutrients. Anorexia needs fast action.

What about food binges and purges – are they a problem?

Bulimia occurs when you gorge on food and then self-induce sickness so as not to put on weight. You effectively lose control over your eating and feel compelled to overeat. You may also use laxatives or diuretics in an effort to get rid of the excess calories. The condition is ten times more common in women than in men. Sufferers tend to simply go on a binge, which can either be planned so that food is pre-bought or spontaneous. Afterwards they tend to feel totally stuffed as well as ashamed and guilty about what they have done and their potential weight gain, so self-inducing sickness is seen as a form of damage limitation.

Who's at risk of bulimia?

Women with low self-esteem are at great risk. Depression and stress can also be a trigger, as can life events such as divorce or death. It can also follow in families, so if you have a close relative who is affected, you are four times more likely to fall prey to it. Women who are overweight or have an element of body dysmorphic disorder in which they believe they are overweight are also prone to this problem.

Is bulimia bad?

Yes, as it leads to both physical and psychological problems. The acid from vomiting erodes your teeth and gives you bad breath. Skin and hair tend to be lacklustre due to the deficiency of vitamins and minerals. Energy tends to be zapped. Constipation is also a common problem, as are irregular periods. Mood swings, low self-esteem, anxiety and tension are common in bulimia. Ironically, the purging activity does not tend to result in a great deal of weight loss, and the person with bulimia tends to be of average or above average weight.

How can these conditions be helped?

As with all mental health conditions, the first step towards treatment is admitting in the first place that there is a problem that needs to be treated. This is the most difficult milestone to overcome. In the event that anorexia has become extremely severe, the individual may be admitted to hospital under a compulsory order if doctors feel that their life is at risk.

In general terms, cognitive-behavioural therapy is the main therapy used to tackle all of these disorders; this approach endeavours to help you overcome the false beliefs and negative thoughts you have about yourself and your body image. It walks you through the journey of how you got to where you are today. It then works on your thought processes so you can walk yourself back to how you were and be happy to be there.

Medication may also be used, and this usually takes the form of SSRI (selective serotonin reuptake inhibitor) antidepressants. This does not mean that you are depressed, although anorexia, bulimia and body dysmorphic disorder can all be the cause or the effect of depression. The SSRI drugs are used for many purposes and are the drugs of first choice in these three conditions.

What does the future hold?

There is no specific cure for any of these disorders, but the same is true of many medical conditions, so don't dismay. Insight into the problem and being on the alert for the signs and symptoms of a relapse are crucial. After pregnancy is a risk time for relapse for all of these conditions.

If you are worried about any form of eating disorder or body dysmorphia, do go and see your doctor. He or she will have dealt with these problems before and is best placed to help you. Although you may feel alone, 'going it alone' is not the way forward – external support is the key to success.

Urinary system

9

Tune in to some basic plumbing problems with this guided tour of what can go wrong with your waterworks.

CYSTITIS

Cystitis can be the bane of a woman's life. It comes from 'cyst' meaning bladder and 'itis', referring to inflammation. Put the two together and you get a problem that besieges some women but comes to most of us at least once in our lifetime. Women get it much more commonly than men because our water pipes are shorter and they lie in closer proximity to our back passages.

Preventative measures

- Don't hold urine – if you've gotta go, you've gotta go.
- Avoid baths as long soaks promote cystitis.
- Wipe from front to back after a bowel movement to prevent cross-contamination.
- Drink lots of fluid. Cranberry juice is thought to be particularly helpful.
- Although it's a passion-killer, pass urine before and after intercourse if possible.
- Don't douche or overcleanse the skin around the vagina and anus.

THE URINARY SYSTEM

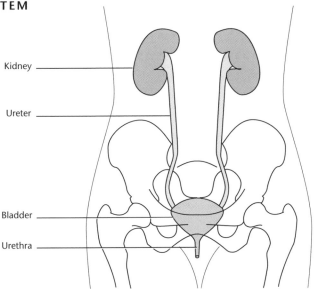

Kidney

Ureter

Bladder

Urethra

169

Who is most likely to get it?

Sexually active women, those who have diabetes, women in the menopause and pregnant women are most likely to suffer.

What are the symptoms?

- There is usually a desire to pass more urine.
- Urination may be painful – it's often described as peeing glass!
- There may be blood in the urine or it may look cloudy.
- You may have flu-like symptoms or fever.
- There may be aches and pains in your back or over your bladder.

Diagnosis This is easy based on the symptoms, so you can usually diagnose it yourself. If, however, you have a lot of blood, are in a lot of pain, have high fever or feel unwell, you should see the doctor. Any symptoms that do not resolve after forty-eight hours also need checking.

Treatments You can treat yourself at home with fluids to try to cleanse the system. Double your daily fluid intake. Water with a half a teaspoon of sodium bicarbonate in helps to neutralise the acid in the urine and so ease the pain. If you aren't a cook and don't have this at home, you can buy a similar substance at the pharmacist.

Antibiotics are necessary if your symptoms are severe or ongoing. Your doctor will usually confirm the infection by testing your urine with a dipstick and then sending the urine to the lab if the diagnosis is in doubt or warrants confirmation.

Problems

Recurrent cystitis can be a problem, and it's often brought on by sex. If this is the case, your doctor may put you on a low dose of an antibiotic taken every night for about ninety days. An alternative is to take it directly after sex. Busy young women who drink caffeine and alcohol and wear skinny jeans or tight pencil skirts and nylons can be very prone. Push your hydration levels, ditch tight clothing in favour of loose garments, buy cotton knickers and buy big!

Follow-up

If you are getting several bouts of cystitis a year, it is worth asking your doctor for an emergency prescription of antibiotics as at this stage you should be confident in diagnosing the condition yourself. If the problem is unrelenting, ask to be referred to a urogynaecologist, who will do further tests to check the flow and function of the kidneys and bladder.

Tip ▌ *Recurrent cystitis may not be a simple urine infection. Discount Chlamydia by getting your doctor to test for it.*

BLADDER CONTROL

Are you controlling your bladder or is it controlling you?

Like it or not, ladies, one in every five of us leak. Incontinence is more common than hay fever in women, and it's twice as common in women as men.

Stress incontinence

This occurs when the pelvic floor is weak, so the scaffolding that supports the bladder is not as effective. As a result, physical activity that increases the pressure in the abdomen causes the bladder to leak. This can occur when you cough, sneeze, laugh or run. This is the most common form.

Urge incontinence

This occurs when the bladder muscle contracts too early, so if you've got to go, you really have got to go! You may generally feel the urge but not have time to get to the toilet.

Overactive bladder

In OAB the bladder seems to be hyperactive, so its nerves and muscles are kicking off uninvited, and you are always in search of a loo. As a rule of thumb, if you are going more than seven times a day or are up twice or more in the night, something is amiss. We call it OAB wet if it's accompanied by incontinence and OAB dry if it isn't.

What's the next step if I seem to be wet?

To regain control, you need to work on the muscles. Physiotherapy can help to distinguish which are which. Imagine you are trying to pick up a marble with your vagina, retain it inside and count to three. It also helps to imagine you are passing urine but the phone rings so you need to stop the flow – the muscles you squeeze are the ones you need to work on. If you do ten repetitions of this three times a day, you may see an improvement in your pelvic floor function in twelve weeks. You can also buy training cones that you can insert and squeeze, training your muscles to keep them in place. These techniques work best for stress incontinence or mixed incontinence.

The bladder usually contracts when it is half full, but we can generally override this desire and hold on. In urge incontinence and OAB, this message does not get through. This is tackled by re-educating the bladder and effectively trying to get you to hold on for longer. Tablets also help as they interfere with the signals going to the bladder that are causing it to contract, i.e. the involuntary signals. Pills are, however, not without their side-effects, dry mouth, constipation and blurred vision being most common.

What causes it in the first place?

Menopause, childbirth, infections, diabetes, age and obesity are all culprits.

Are tests needed?

You may not need any tests if the diagnosis is straightforward. However, if you see a specialist, he or she will order urine tests, bladder flow studies and scans.

Can't I have an operation?

Conservative management, i.e. avoiding the knife, is the name of the game. Stress incontinence may be helped by a TVT – a tension-free vaginal tape – to tighten things up. A more formal strengthening of the pelvic floor known as a colposuspension may be an option if all else fails. Nerve stimulation operations are recommended for suitable women with urge incontinence when bladder drill and pills have failed.

Tip *Start your pelvic floor exercises in pregnancy to prevent future problems.*

Pitfalls *Avoid squeezing the pelvic floor inappropriately just because you don't know your anatomy.*

KIDNEY STONES

There are two words to describe kidney stones – 'downright' and 'painful'. Pain usually comes on suddenly in the sides or the back. You want to pass urine more often, there may be blood in your urine, it can hurt to go to the toilet, and you may have a fever.

Who is most likely to get kidney stones?

Men are more prone, but six in every hundred women will get one at some point. They generally occur between the ages of thirty and sixty. You're more likely to suffer if you have high blood pressure, a family member has had them or you are white skinned. We tend to suffer more if we don't drink a lot of water, take diuretic pills or too much calcium or vitamin C, drink too much alcohol or are prone to kidney infections. If you are abusing laxatives or adhering to faddy high-protein diets, you're also at risk. If you have previously had a kidney stone, there's a 50/50 chance of developing another within five years.

So what are they?

Your kidneys are a filter system that ultrafiltrates your blood and rids the body of waste products via the urine. Occasionally, some of this waste produce may be in the form of crystals or grains. If these become large, they form a stone and can get caught in our water pipes.

Are they a problem?

Many kidney stones pass easily. But if their diameter is greater than 5mm, they are destined to cause mischief. They can cause problems within the kidney or inside the water pipes, which results in blockage. As in a sewage system, extra pressure is then put on the mains – the kidney – and the outflow is limited. This can result in contamination, giving rise to infection.

How would I know I had a stone?

When a stone gets stuck in the water pipe, there can be very severe pain usually originating in the lower back or side between the pelvis and ribs. This is often described as colic because it tends to come in peaks and troughs, and is often said to be far more painful than labour! You may find it difficult to go to the toilet, and your urine may be cloudy or bloody. You may also have the sweats and feel generally off form.

What does the doctor do?

You will be asked to give a urine sample, which will usually test positive for blood from the stone itself and often from infection. Your blood will be checked to establish your baseline kidney function and see whether you have excesses of compounds in your blood that might precipitate stones – such as uric acid (common in gout) or excessive calcium (common in ladies who take calcium supplements).

An X-ray will show stones made of calcium, which account for 90 per cent of kidney stones, but will miss others made from different substances. In this situation, a dye is injected into the veins and followed as it passes through the kidney – this will show up blockages in the system. CT (computed tomography) scans may also be used. Ultrasound scans aren't great at showing up stones, so a normal scan doesn't necessarily rule a stone out.

Can I get rid of a stone?

A stone can be as small as a grain of pepper or as big as a plum. Most small stones pass in the urine after about seventy-two hours. Your doctor may, rather oddly, ask you to sieve your urine to collect any grit. Stones as big as 9mm may pass, but they often need to be helped out. Shock waves can be used externally, which smash the stone into smaller pieces that are easier to excrete. Or a telescope can be inserted into the water pipe or kidney, and the stone is broken up and then removed.

Do I always need hospital treatment or can my family doctor manage it?

Not all stones require hospital intervention – it depends on the site, size and symptoms. Small stones may be managed at home by adequate pain relief, rest, antibiotics to cover for infection and rehydration with two to three litres of water. These stones generally pass after a few days without incident. Any lingering pain or problems with urination demand referral to hospital to establish the diagnosis and treatment.

What if I think I've got a stone?

If you have a family history of stones, it's worth mentioning to the doctor if any urinary symptoms crop up. Try to avoid the drugs and triggers mentioned above to prevent stones forming or existing ones worsening. A quick urine test can decide if antibiotics are required or a stone is suspected. If it is, you would be daft to leave the doctor's without any pain relief as stones can become very painful very quickly. If you are known to have a stone, have an action plan of what to do if it starts to play up. Generally, it's fluids, antibiotics and pain relief that are the urgent requirement, plus or minus a urologist – I usually give my patients a letter so they can queue jump in the emergency room as the diagnosis has already been established.

Tips
Excessive amounts of rhubarb and caffeine trigger kidney stones, as may exercising intensely in a warm climate. Drink enough water to make sure your urine is pale and clear – any deviation towards a barley-water shade smacks of dehydration. Two litres plus of fluid a day can prevent further attacks.

If you do pass a stone at home, then, silly as it sounds, keep it so your doctor can have it analysed. The type of stone may be the key to why you developed it in the first instance.

Don't overdo vitamin C supplements as this can result in kidney stones.

Neurology

10

Worried about headaches, shakes and muscular twitches?
The neurology section will teach you more.

WHAT'S IN A HEADACHE?

Headache is one of the most common pains to occur in the body. Headaches can occur because we worry, and they can in turn cause us to worry. It is, however, true to say that the vast majority of headaches are due to straightforward causes, so you don't need to worry!

Tension headache

These are very common, and most women will have experienced one if not many. We are twice as likely to suffer as men. Indeed, tension headaches can occur once to twice a month in some women, and about three in a hundred women have one almost every day. In these headaches, there is a band of tightness or pressure around the forehead, neck or back of the head. They tend to come and go and are not accompanied by any other symptoms such as dizziness. By and large, you work though a tension headache. It can last for minutes or days but does not affect sleep. They can be brought on by stress, poor posture, tiredness, depression or fatigue.

Migraine

The link between migraine and the menstrual cycle is long established. Before puberty, girls equal boys in the migraine stakes, but during the childbearing years women outnumber men by three to one. Migraine is due to a spasm of the blood vessels leading to the brain and the subsequent release of chemicals. Typically, a migraine feels like a throbbing pain or a pulsation. You may feel nauseous or vomit. You can feel numb or weak down one side. Vision can be blurred, smells and sounds enhanced. The sufferer often shuns light and needs to lie down in a darkened room. Sometimes you get a warning and can feel it coming on. This is called an aura and often results in the sufferer experiencing visual symptoms before the pain sets in.

Cluster headache

This isn't very common and generally tends to affect men, so most women are spared. Pain is typically one-sided, severe and localised to one eye. It occurs in clusters over time and no one knows what causes it.

Other causes of headache

Sinus problems, jaw dysfunction, tooth grinding at night, ear infections, dehydration and eye strain can all be a cause. Rarely, a headache is due to a brain tumour, haemorrhage or meningitis.

Do some detective work by making a headache diary

If you are experiencing headaches, make a symptoms diary, scoring the severity out of ten and noting down any associated features or triggers. This helps the doctor to get a clear picture of what is going on in the consultation and also in your head!

Treatment Tension-type headaches can be treated with over-the-counter painkillers such as ibuprofen and paracetamol if they are severe. Relaxation therapy and exercise can also help. Acupuncture and craniosacral massage are alternative treatments that work well for stress and tension headaches, so don't be afraid to try alternatives to tablet popping. Assess your work station set up in the office or at home if you tend to use your computer a lot, and make sure that your posture when you sit to work isn't causing your headache. Physiotherapy may help to work on your core muscles and posture, and reduce any muscle spasm.

Look at your diet and pick out any triggers. Watch out for blood sugar crashes (so missing breakfast and going on faddy diets are a no-no), caffeine overloads and Chinese takeaways that contain MSG (monosodium glutamate), all of which can contribute to headache.

Drink at least a litre (two pints) of water a day. Air-conditioned offices and central heating contribute to dehydration – you only have to watch the house plants wilt to see what harm it does. And it goes without saying that you should ban the booze if you want to be headache-free.

WHEN IS MY HEADACHE A MIGRAINE?

As many as one in four of us will suffer from a migraine at some point in our lives, and in 90 per cent of cases this will happen before we hit forty. A migraine is no ordinary headache – it doesn't come and go like the tension type, and it effectively announces its arrival to prepare you for the pain. We call this the prodromal phase, and sufferers tend to feel tired and cranky.

In about 15 per cent of sufferers, this is followed by five minutes to a full hour of what is known as an aura. This may take the form of spots in the vision or zigzag lines appearing, along with confusion, disorientation, pins and needles or even fainting. Coordination and speech may be disturbed, so the individual almost seems drunk. This heralds the onset of the headache.

Generally, the headache pain is throbbing and extreme, and the sufferer feels very nauseous, often vomiting as well. Light, sounds and smells may also seem exaggerated, so you will want to lie down in a quiet room. This can go on for between three hours and three days – it's very variable.

The attack the generally fades away, but you are left with a sensation of tiredness and almost a hangover effect from the event; it may take several days to feel normal again. So, as you can see, migraine is no ordinary headache – in fact it can be an extraordinary menace.

What's the diagnosis doctor?

By and large, migraine is easy enough to diagnose without any further tests. The key is in the sequence of events, which is why it is helpful to make a headache diary. Migraine follows a particular pattern of severe pain, nausea often accompanied by vomiting and increased sensitivity. We call it 'common' migraine if it is not accompanied by the aura phase, and 'migraine with aura' if it is.

The condition often runs in families, so tell the doctor if Mum or Auntie May was a migraine suffer. And migraine tends to strike in attacks. Tension headache tends simply to develop and disappear without any significant upset to the system. You could handle a cocktail party with a tension headache, but you wouldn't get past the first canapé with a migraine. If your doctor does diagnose migraine, he or she can only give you the ammunition to deal with it, but it is up to you to wage the war.

Tactics

Have treatment to deal with a migraine attack on you at all times. This can range from over-the-counter migraine treatments to prescription treatments aimed directly at the chemicals involved in a migraine attack.

Ideally, you need something to kill pain and to prevent nausea, which is the usual combination in over-the-counter packs. Simple paracetamol and aspirin work well, but severe migraine often needs more. Your doctor can give you a pill, a wafer-type medicine that melts in your mouth or a spray to squirt up your nose. This group of medicines are called called triptans, and they affect a chemical in the brain thought to be involved in migraine. They generally prevent or stop a migraine attack. You can buy sumatriptan over the counter in the UK, without a prescription, but most of the medicines are only available via prescription.

Sadly, they don't work for everyone, but if you have tried one type and failed, it is worth trying another. If they do work, however, they can literally be life-changing as they can abate an attack in minutes.

Recurrent offenders

If you suffer from more than two migraine attacks a month that stop work or socialisation, if you have very severe attacks or you have attacks that don't respond to treatment, you should consider taking something on a regular basis. These medicines often take three months to become effective, and you are usually advised to take them for a minimum of six months – it is very much trial and error as you need to see what happens in terms of your migraine when you come off them.

Old-fashioned beta-blockers can be used and tend to work well in preventing migraine, but we're not sure exactly how they work. These medications are also used for blood pressure and anxiety, so don't think your doctor has got the prescription wrong if you get one for these – beta-blockers are multipurpose. Unfortunately, people with asthma can't take them, and in terms of side-effects tiredness and cold hands and feet are often reported.

Amitriptyline is an old fashioned antidepressant that has been found to be helpful in preventing migraine. The newer SSRI (selective serotonin reuptake inhibitor) antidepressants such as citalopram can also be used in small doses as a preventative. Other drugs called pizotifen and methisergide can be given on a daily basis to prevent migraine, but they do have problems of weight gain and drowsiness. One in three people who take them, however, report a decrease in both the severity and the frequency of attacks.

Topirimate, sodium valproate (valproic acid) and gabapentin are all antiepilepsy drugs that are also used in the prevention of migraine. In addition, magnesium supplements in your diet have been shown to help with the prevention of attacks.

Take it seriously

If you have migraine, take it seriously as otherwise it can take you over – the World Health Organization has ranked it in their top twenty causes of disability in terms of years of healthy life lost because of it. It stands to reason that you can be wiped out by an attack for up to three days. It is also thought that depression is at least twice as common in migraine sufferers than average.

Question the diagnosis

If you really feel you are not a migraineur (that's the term for a migraine sufferer), ask your doctor to refer you to a migraine clinic for a further assessment. This is also a good option if you feel that 'the drugs don't work' and that you are getting nowhere in terms of medical management. Don't accept a new diagnosis of migraine if you are over forty – ask to see a neurologist as the vast majority of suffers succumb before this milestone and there could be something else wrong.

The menstrual cycle, menopause and the pill

Fifty per cent of migraine sufferers have problems related to their menstrual cycle, and seem to run into problems around the menopause. The pill can cause migraine too, and individuals who experience migraine with aura, i.e. migraine with an associated blurring of vision, flashing lights or tunnel vision, should NOT take a contraceptive pill containing oestrogen and progesterone as it may increase their risk of a stroke.

Tip Think you have migraine? Don't self-diagnose; let the doctor do the work.

Myth Pregnancy makes migraine worse. No – in fact, two thirds of migraine sufferers improve during pregnancy.

Pitfall Taking regular pain relief for headaches can actually and paradoxically cause headaches in the long term. We call this analgesia headache. Beware – this is particularly true of drugs that contain caffeine and codeine, so always read the label.

Complete this diary and take the results with you when visiting your pharmacist, doctor or nurse.

HEADACHE/MIGRAINE DIARY

Date and day of week	Time attack starts	Time attack ends	Severity 1 to 10	Feel sick Yes / No	Vomit Yes / No	Medication taken	Effective Yes / No	Period Yes / No

DO YOU TREMOR, TREMBLE OR QUIVER?

We all shake a little when we are scared; it's a natural reaction brought on by adrenaline. But tremor, as we medics call it, can occur for other reasons. We define it as an unintentional, uncontrollable shaking of part of the body. It tends to be a symptom or sign of an underlying condition or an exaggeration of a normal bodily reaction.

Keep it in the family

Tremor can run in families. It's thought to result from a faulty gene, and if one of your parents has it there's a 50/50 chance you'll be troubled too. This type of tremor is benign, which means it's not due to an underlying sinister disease.

How do you diagnose a tremor?

Most people notice their symptoms and many try to hide them. People usually end up at the doctor's for two reasons. First, they are worried it might be the sign of an underlying disorder, the most common concern being Parkinson's disease. Second, they may be unable to carry out normal daily activities.

To check yourself for tremor, hold your hands out in front of you at shoulder height, palms down. Ask someone to place a piece of A4 paper on them – if you have a significant tremor, the paper will start to shake and will eventually fall off. It's also obvious if you try to write as your script will be very spidery. Most tremors occur in the hands but they can occur anywhere, for example the head, arms, legs or even voice. There are over twenty different types of tremor. The doctor can usually work out the cause by examining you. Occasionally, you may need blood and urine tests or a visit to a neurologist and a scan to rule out underlying disorders.

Is something radically wrong?

In those who are young and healthy, there is often no serious underlying cause, and it may be familial. But it can also occur as a one-off, and it's generally accepted that it's due to an alteration in signals to the cerebellum. This is the part of the brain that deals with balance and coordination, so it's the area of the brain that is affected when you are drunk and that enables you to play the piano. This type of tremor is called essential tremor. Essential means there is no specific underlying cause for it. This is the most common cause of tremor seen in doctors' clinics.

Tremor can also occur because of an overactive thyroid gland, low blood sugar, stimulants such as speed and cocaine, diet pills, asthma drugs such as salbutamol (albuterol), or theophylline, alcohol withdrawal, mercury poisoning, liver disease and too much caffeine. Significant neurological problems, including multiple sclerosis and Parkinson's disease, are also a cause, as is stroke. With serious conditions like these, there are typically signs of the underlying disorder too – a stroke-type tremor may be associated with weakness, and a multiple sclerosis-type tremor with blurred vision.

Can it be cured?

Tremor as a side-effect of drugs, alcohol or diet can be cured by eliminating the contributing factor. Tremor due to an underlying disease may be improved by improving the underlying condition. Benign essential tremor cannot be cured and unfortunately tends to get worse. The goal is to treat the symptoms and eliminate the trigger factors.

Do the drugs work?

There's about a 50/50 chance of improvement with drug treatment alone. Propranolol, used for migraine, anxiety and high blood pressure, has a role here. It's the best-tolerated drug so probably the one you should try first. It can cause tiredness and cold feet and hands, and is unsuitable for asthmatics. Primidone and topirimate can also be trialled, but the former may affect mood and concentration, and the latter cause weight loss and appetite suppression. Neither drug gives rise to a rapid response. Botox is another option but it can have the unfortunate side-effect of hand paralysis.

At home on the sofa, how can I self-diagnose a good tremor from a bad one?

Essential tremor tends to start in one hand and then progress to involve the other. It may be intermittent to start with but then develop to become constant. It does not occur during sleep and is often improved by alcohol or rest. The tremor of Parkinson's disease occurs at rest and is described as pill rolling – it's like someone rolling a cigarette between their thumb and index finger. It's classic to the trained eye. Tremor caused by stroke or multiple sclerosis is often termed intention tremor – classically, you go to pick up a coin on the ground and overshoot it.

How common is this problem?

It is far more common than you may think, though it's difficult to get accurate statistics as many people won't visit their doctor. An estimated 4 to 5 per cent of the forty to sixty year age group suffer from some form of tremor, and over 5 per cent of the over sixties suffer from the shakes. So it's not confined to an older population, and it favours neither men nor women.

When should I seek help?

Even if you have had your tremor for years, see your doctor. There may be no cure, but treatment may improve your symptoms and allow you a better quality of life. Many people who suffer from essential tremor are ashamed and isolated, and often shun social activities. People worry others may think they have an alcohol problem or are disabled by some form of neurological disorder. So it's really important both to understand your problem yourself and to be able to explain it to others. The other reason for seeing your doctor is that your tremor, especially if it has come on only recently, may be the sign of an underlying problem that needs attention. Although most shakes aren't sinister, they still warrant seeing the doctor, if only to document the fact in your records.

Tips

▌ *Train your tremor-free hand to do as many things as possible, for example write.*

▌ *Steady your shaky hand with your less shaky hand as it will make fine movements easier.*

▌ *Use travel mugs with lids, and carry straws with you for taking beverages in public. Eat finger food platters if out to lunch so you can avoid cutlery nightmares. And steer clear of plastic cutlery – heavy knives and forks will make you shake less.*

▌ *Keep your elbows close to your body as your quiver will be less obvious.*

▌ *Use an electric toothbrush as it's easier to control.*

▌ *Print rather than use joined-up writing.*

MULTIPLE SCLEROSIS

Most of us have heard of this but what exactly is it? Well, it occurs when your body starts to reject the protective coating called myelin that surrounds your nerves. This is referred to as demyelination. Multiple sclerosis – MS – is a disease that is twice as common in women and usually occurs between the ages of twenty and forty. Like many diseases it can't be cured, but there are a variety of drugs that help to control the symptoms.

So how would I know I had it?

One in four women who develop MS will initially seek medical advice for an eye problem. This usually takes the form of pain or blurred vision in one eye, and occasionally double vision or colour vision problems. Some women experience pain, sensitive burning skin, numbness or pins and needles all over their body. Coordination may be a problem, with a sensation of dizziness, wobbliness or the spins. You may become very tired or forgetful or have difficulty concentrating, and your mood may go up and down. Your waterworks may be affected – your bladder may be overactive so you're in the bathroom every minute, or your bladder doesn't feel as if it's emptying properly. The same is true for your bowels – they can block up or give you the runs. So the symptoms can be very varied.

How do you contract it?

You don't contract it or pass it on – it's an autoimmune disease. These are the diseases where your body starts to reject its own parts, a bit like a kidney transplant failing to work because your body is mounting an immune response against it. Autoimmune diseases are far more common in women. Your immune system causes the insulating myelin coating around your nervous system to become inflamed so the nerve impulses don't get passed through. It's a bit like an electric cable not being insulated because it's got wet. When the inflammation passes, the nerves start to fire again and the symptoms disappear.

What's the switch that starts the process?

We don't fully know. A viral infection may trigger the response, and it's more common in people who have first-degree relatives with MS and the further you live from the equator. Environment is thought to have an impact as, bizarrely, European Gypsies, Eskimos and certain African tribes rarely develop it.

It can be diagnosed on a blood test though, can't it?

No. It's tested for by an MRI (magnetic resonance imaging) scan, which can show areas of scarring or inflammation in the myelin. It can also be tested for with a lumbar puncture, where a needle is passed into the base of your spine to analyse your spinal fluid – as for meningitis. Visual evoked potential tests can also be carried out, which measure nerve conduction impulses in the visual pathway.

Is it bad news if I have it?

It's a difficult diagnosis for a doctor to make as patients have a preconceived idea of its severity. The reality is that 90 per cent of women have the type of MS that relapses and remits. This means they experience symptoms for two to six weeks and these then settle – they either go away or ease to the point they are barely perceptible. Then another attack strikes in a year or so. The problem is that the more attacks you have, the more damage it does to the nerves, and slowly the symptoms don't recover as the nerves become scarred.

Two out of every three sufferers will progress to what is called secondary progressive MS by about the fifteenth anniversary of their first attack. By the twenty-fifth anniversary, this figure is close to 90 per cent. Ten per cent of suffers do not have any relapses, and their symptoms are continuous and more progressive. This is called primary progressive MS and is much rarer. A number of people have what is called benign MS, whereby you get a full recovery after an attack, very few relapses and no permanent damage. This probably accounts for 5 to 10 per cent of cases. The bottom line is that the more frequent the attacks and the more severe their aftermath, the worse you fare.

What about pregnancy?

MS is diagnosed in women of childbearing age more frequently than in any other group. The condition itself does not affect your fertility, but the drugs used to treat it may affect your periods or damage an unborn baby. Otherwise your pregnancy, labour and delivery should be the same as any other mother's, and your baby won't have any increased risk of complications. The frequency of attacks seems to decrease during pregnancy, but they increase again in the first three months after delivery. This is thought to be an effect of the female hormone oestrogen on your immune system.

So there's no cure but are there treatments?

Yes, different things can be taken at different stages of the disease. Steroids are the mainstay of treatment to tackle the 'acute' phases and relapses. It makes sense to hit the inflammation hard by giving high doses through the veins for three days, followed by oral steroids.

The next step is disease-modifying therapy, which aims to make relapses less frequent and less severe, so it's damage limitation. Drugs that modify your immune response include beta-interferon, glatiramer acetate and natalizumab. They don't cure it, but they do help prevent relapses and may slow its progress. The beta-interferons and natalizumab modify your immune response, and glatiramer acetate mimics the effects of the protein in myelin. Your neurologist will discuss which will work best for you. They are often self-administered via injection, like insulin.

Who fares best with MS?

The course of MS is difficult to forecast. Good outcomes are seen in women, those who have their first attack before the age of forty, those who recover totally from the first attack and those who have a long gap between the first and second strikes of MS. And the fewer the signs on a brain scan, the better the outcome.

What should I do if I'm worried about MS?

You are likely to be worried if you have a relation with it – 20 per cent of sufferers have an affected relative. Your risk if you have a first-degree relative affected is about 1 per cent; otherwise, it's one in a thousand. Talk to your doctor about your symptoms, their frequency and duration. Let the doctor know what you are worried about, and together you can decide whether you need reassurance or referral to a neurologist. Remember, your doctor can't rule out MS on a blood test.

Food for thought

One third of women diagnosed with MS are still at work and enjoying an active life fifteen years later.

Gastro-intestinal

11

Good gut, bad gut – there's lots of it inside you to summon up trouble. Find out more about your gut and how to love it.

THE DIGESTIVE SYSTEM

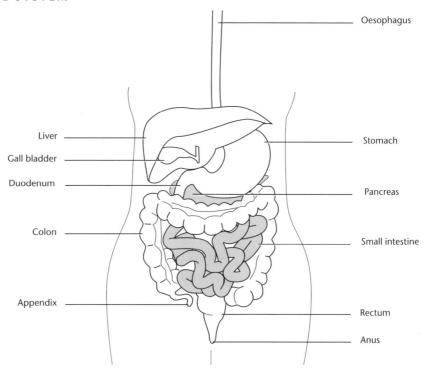

Oesophagus

Liver

Gall bladder

Duodenum

Colon

Appendix

Stomach

Pancreas

Small intestine

Rectum

Anus

CONSTIPATION

Constipation is a curse. It leaves us feeling sluggish, bloated, heavy and uncomfortable. Irrespective of the symptoms, constipation in its own right is the root of many evils.

Why do we clog up with constipation?

- Pregnancy
- Dehydration
- Illness
- Medication such as codeine

- Calcium and iron supplements
- Poor dietary fibre intake
- Immobility
- Irritable bowel syndrome

What's so good about fibre?

Fibre helps to form soft bulky motions that pass easily though the gut. The food we eat has to travel nine metres before it finds its way into our toilet bowl. Fibre makes this transit easier by making the bowel motions large enough to stimulate contractions in the gut muscle and smooth enough to glide easily though the gut when it contracts. If you aren't a fibre fan, introduce it gradually as otherwise it will give you tummy cramps. Water is also essential as it goes hand in hand with fibre.

There are two types of fibre. Soluble fibre is broken down partially in our guts to give us energy, produce gas and make our stools bulky. Fruit, vegetables, seeds, oats, barley, peas and beans all belong to this category. Fruit and veg with skins and pips form insoluble fibre, as do brown rice and whole grains. These fibres don't break down as easily so hold water, adding weight to our stools. They help speed up the transport of other substances in the gut and push them through, and are often referred to as nature's broom as they help clear out the gut.

If you are constipated and eat little fibre, do the double high five rule, meaning that instead of five a day, do ten fruit and veg a day for the first forty-eight hours. The fibre content combined with drinking lots of water should get you started.

Laxatives

These play a role in unblocking the system, but their regular use is not advised as most constipation can be cleared with diet, fibre and fluid. Laxatives work by making the stool easier to pass by softening it or bulking, or by stimulating the bowel to contract. Tell the doctor if you have been using laxatives. Prunes and figs are natural laxatives and have the added benefit of being part of your five a day. Exercise helps too!

Answer the call

Women are often too embarrassed to pass a bowel motion in a public toilet. This can be a particular problem in the workplace, but is nothing to be ashamed of. Storing up bowel motions until you get home is a common cause of constipation.

Tips ▌ *The bowels should ideally be opened daily. We are all different, but your goals should be: Go more than twice a week. Go without straining. Go with a soft stool. Go without laxatives.*

BLEEDING FROM THE BACK PASSAGE

Nothing scares a person more than the sight of blood from the back passage. It generally splats onto the toilet bowl and appears on the toilet paper or mixed in with the stool. Although you can think of every reason under the sun for not seeking medical advice about it, you simply must.

Anticipate questions

Doctors are going to ask you about constipation and straining to open your bowels. They will want to know if the blood is fresh, i.e. bright red, or seems old. Tell them about changes in the pattern of your bowel habit, diarrhoea, slime, mucus, flatulence or incontinence, and volunteer information about bowel problems in the family. Mention whether you have lost weight or had stomach pain.

Let's talk piles

Bleeding from the back passage is generally due to either trauma or haemorrhoids – piles – which are just varicose veins of the anus and rectum. Fifty per cent of the population have these by the time they are fifty. Women tend to suffer during pregnancy, but this usually resolves after the birth. Constipation, straining, old age and anal intercourse may contribute.

How do I know I've got them? Often you don't, and the first sign is when fresh blood appears in the toilet. If the haemorrhoids poke out, you may feel a sore, hard lump. The doctor can confirm the diagnosis with an examination of the back passage.

Treatment If you are constipated, you need to be unclogged as straining causes haemorrhoid hell. Piles can be treated by creams applied externally and suppositories applied internally. These products are available over the counter, although the doctor may need to give you a stronger treatment on prescription. When the swollen haemorrhoid shrinks, the area of skin overlying it tends to hang as a skin tag. This can give the feeling of a ruffle around the back passage and may become irritated when you are cleaning yourself.

A visit to a surgeon is only necessary if the piles are persistent, problematic or protruding. They tend to look and feel like a bunch of grapes. Banding involves placing an elastic band around the base of the haemorrhoid so the blood supply is cut off. It's left there for seven days so that the haemorrhoid dies and falls off. Sclerotherapy involves injecting a chemical directly into the haemorrhoid, which makes it shrivel up. Haemorrhoidectomy involves cutting out the haemorrhoids and stretching the back passage. The haemorrhoids are less likely to come back after this radical removal, but it's a sore procedure – you'll need at least a week off work.

Other causes of bleeding from the bottom

Any skin irritation or infection that results in itching or scratching can cause bleeding. If the bleeding is associated with diarrhoea, mucus or a change in bowel habit, colitis needs to be ruled out. Anorectal cancers or polyps, and tears or cracks (fissures) in the lining of the back passage can result in bleeding, as can straining if you are constipated.

Make fibre your friend

Eat lots of fibre and drink lots of fluid to prevent constipation – this is key in keeping haemorrhoids at bay. Fibre is the scaffolding that holds a plant together. We can chew it, swallow it and stuff our bellies with it, but we usually do not digest it. Problem? No – it's actually helpful in practical terms. It helps the gut work better, promotes good bacteria, softens our bowel motions, helps us lower our cholesterol and fights against cancer of the colon. Fruit, veg, seeds and grains all contain fibre, so get grazing!

Tip *If you piles are pestering you, wrap some ice in a tea towel and sit on it for twenty minutes.*

Myth *If you ignore piles, they go away. No – they usually become worse and a task to treat.*

ITCHY BOTTOM

You know how doctors like to use fancy names for things? Well, we call this pruritis ani. Although it sounds scientific, it simply means an itchy rear end. It's incredibly common, and undeniably embarrassing.

So what's making you scratch?

It could be an anal fissure, a thrush infection, dermatitis, piles, scabies or even worms. It might also be impossible to work out what's causing it. Typically, scabies and worms tend to be more scratchy by night. Piles or a fissure can cause bleeding. And skin problems like contact dermatitis or seborrhoeic eczema tend to crop up at other sites on the body as well.

Can't I just treat it myself and not go to the doctor?

No, an itchy bottom symptom that is ongoing needs attention. Even with your best gymnastic efforts using make-up mirrors, you cannot really view things with clarity. So book an appointment with your doctor and prime yourself for some searching questions and probably an examination.

What's next?

Talk to the doctor. They need to know how long it has been going on for, when it's worse and what drives it. Also mention any treatments you have tried, even if they seem insignificant. You are likely to be asked about your bowel habit and any bleeding or change in the motions. Do you feel well? Are you stressed or worried?

Checks

You may need to have your bottom looked at. By looking, the doctor can often diagnose things like eczema. If you have symptoms suggesting haemorrhoids, you may need an examination of your back passage in which the doctor inserts a gloved finger to check for any abnormalities. A swab is likely to be taken if it looks like there is an infection, for example thrush. Blood tests for diabetes, liver and kidney function, thyroid gland and iron level may be ordered.

How can I help?

If you have long nails, they need the chop. When drying your rear end, use soft loo paper after going to the bathroom and dry the area with a hairdryer after a bath or shower. If you need to use a towel, pat, don't rub. Throw out the thongs – they are the enemy! Get the cotton granny knickers on and avoid nylons and any tight clothing. Wash the area using aqueous cream as a soap substitute and avoid bath salts and perfumed soaps. Stop all other cream lotions and potions going onto the area unless they have been prescribed by the doctor.

Barrier creams that are used for nappy rash can sometimes help. If the area is inflamed, steroid ointments such as low-strength hydrocortisone 1 per cent can be used. The doctor can treat any thrush or bacteria that may be found. If worms are the problem, over-the-counter antiworming pills will kill them – you may spot worms as little white strings in your motions, which you could have picked up from your kids' sand pit. Scabies generally tends to be scratchy all over and is again treated by a trip to the pharmacist. If night-time scratching is a real problem, a sedative antihistamine can work magic at bedtime in breaking the itch–scratch cycle. Ditch anything in the diet that you may suspect as a trigger, for example beer, caffeine, spices and often citrus fruits or tomatoes.

If you are still itchy and scratchy after three to four weeks despite treatment and tests, your doctor is likely to refer you to a specialist, either a skin specialist or a colorectal surgeon, who is essentially a bottom doctor. If you have been given a steroid treatment, don't use this for longer than fourteen days in this area as it can lead to thinning of the skin, and although you may think it is helping, it's probably making things much worse.

Tip ▌ *Don't overclean the area as, paradoxically, it often makes the condition worse.*

IBS

Irritable bowel syndrome – IBS – is an incredibly common syndrome affecting the gut. We have metres and metres of gut in our bellies, enough in fact to cover a whole tennis court, so when it becomes irritated, it really lets us know.

Who gets it?

One in five of us will get this at some stage of our lives. Women are twice as likely as men to be sufferers. So, statistically, that means it could easily be you.

What are the symptoms?

You'll have pain and discomfort in your abdomen. This tends to come and go and often gets better after you have passed a bowel motion. Bloating also occurs on and off, and most sufferers would describe themselves as 'windy'. Bowel motions can be fast and furious or very sluggish. The size of the motions can change too, to rabbit-poo type or a slimy, mushy stool like a baby's.

BE WARNED, blood is never a symptom of IBS, and the pain and discomfort of IBS does not cause disturbed sleep.

Why does it happen?

Nobody really knows why, but for some reason the bowel becomes irritated and goes into spasm. So, imagining the metres and metres of muscular tube in your belly, the muscle suddenly goes into spasm and voilà, depending on where it squeezes, it causes a burst of diarrhoea or constipation with associated wind and bloatedness. This gives an understanding of why this was previously called 'spastic colon'.

So should I head to the doctor?

Any sudden change in bowel habit needs checking by the doctor. But if you leave the doctors without being offered any tests, don't feel you are being fobbed off as there are no tests for IBS. Occasionally, we have to do tests to rule out other conditions, so you might be asked to provide a blood, stool or urine sample. If your symptoms don't sound like IBS or if they are new symptoms and you are over forty-five, it is likely that

197

you will be referred to a specialist, called a gastroenterologist, for further tests.

Lactose intolerance may be the cause for IBS-type symptoms. This is due to the inability to break down lactose, the sugar found in milk. This condition is far more common in native Americans than Western Europeans. We start life with a lot of the enzyme that breaks down milk sugar, but as time goes on we tend to be less able to digest it and hence we get cramp, flatulence and diarrhoea on ingesting it in, for example, milk and butter, as well as processed foods such as cakes and peanut butter.

How can I help it myself?

I always advise my patients to keep a food/symptom diary for fourteen days. This helps to link triggers such as stress or certain food types to flare-ups in the condition. The

SYMPTOMS CHECKLIST – ARE YOU SUFFERING FROM IBS?

Complete the following questions and take the results with you when visiting your pharmacist, doctor or nurse. It will help them to identify whether the symptoms are due to IBS.

Do you suffer from abdominal spasms / cramps / pain?	Yes/No
Do you suffer from bloating?	Yes/No
Do you suffer from constipation?	Yes/No
Do you suffer from anxiety or depression?	Yes/No
Are you suffering from diarrhoea?	Yes/No
Have you noticed mucus in your stools?	Yes/No
Have you noticed blood in your stools?	Yes/No
List any other possible symptoms that you have been experiencing.	

most common culprits that appear on food diaries are coffee, fizzy drinks, in particular diet drinks, spicy foods, alcohol, processed or fatty foods and white bread. Stress is also hugely significant.

The bacterial status of your gut is also a factor, as we see IBS occurring after a gastrointestinal infection in about one in six cases. Antibiotics can cause problems as they kill the good bacteria in the gut and can give rise to an IBS-type syndrome.

What to do?

Look at your eating habits and adapt them according to your trigger list. Try to eat regular meals and avoid processed foods. If you need to take antibiotics, it'll do you no harm at all to take probiotic drinks or yoghurts afterwards to give you back your good bacteria. Take precautions when you travel to avoid travellers' diarrhoea.

Medicines

The aim of the game is to damp down the symptoms.

Antispasmodics These calm down the gut spasm so can help with gas, distension, diarrhoea, constipation and pain. There are a few types, all of which work slightly differently, so if one doesn't do the trick, others might. It is best to use these on a regular basis for a week when the symptoms flare so you can break the cycle.

Constipation and diarrhoea For those with IBS that blocks them up, using soluble fibre will help. Diarrhoea-dominant IBS? Antidiarrhoeal medicine, for example loperamide, on an as-needed basis for flare-ups is what you need. Beware though, as overuse will block you up!

Antidepressants Patients often become indignant at this suggestion, but although these medicines are named 'antidepressant', what they are antidepressing is your gut and not you. We often use them for chronic problems like back pain or headache, and they really do have a place in treatment.

Other therapies Acupuncture and hypnotherapy have also been used with success, and cognitive-behavioural therapy can help as well.

INDIGESTION

Most of us are familiar with indigestion. But doctors of course choose to use a different word, so we call it dyspepsia – our code word for heartburn.

What are the symptoms?

Generally, you will get discomfort around the bottom of the breast bone or in the throat and neck. You may belch, feel bloated or nauseous and get a bad taste in your mouth or a sensation of burning or pressure in your chest or throat.

What triggers it?

Stress; alcohol; spicy foods; anti-inflammatory tablets, for example ibuprofen, iron or calcium supplements; cigarettes; eating large meals, especially late at night, and eating quickly.

What's happening in indigestion?

It's often a combination of stomach acid and stomach mechanics. We have acid in our stomachs to help digest food; if we have too much or if it finds its way out of the stomach, this can cause problems. Gastritis and oesophagitis can occur whereby the lining of the stomach or the food pipe becomes inflamed, and an ulcer can occur where there is actually a hole in the lining of the gut. Put simply, gastritis is a bit like stripping paint from a wall, whereas an ulcer is like drilling into it. Understandably, one damages the wall more than the other!

What's reflux?

Gastro-oesophageal reflux occurs when acid finds its way from the stomach into the oesophagus. It's like trying to exit through an 'in' door. Reflux can also occur if you have a hiatus hernia, where a portion of the stomach pokes into the chest through the diaphragm –the breathing muscle that separates the chest cage from the abdomen. Although this sounds serious, it's actually relatively common.

Is is appropriate to go to the doctor with indigestion?

If you only have indigestion on and off, you should be able to manage it yourself by modifying your lifestyle and taking antacids as needed to neutralise the stomach acid. If your symptoms are severe, constant, new or unusual, see your doctor.

Treatments Your doctor may prescribe medication to suppress acid. People often worry that this is a bad thing, but in fact this acid is not essential for digestion. Older-style tablets work to block histamine receptors that are involved in acid production. Newer ones called proton pump inhibitors disable the acid pump. These work best, but they are only available on prescription.

Tests Some of us – 50 per cent of women over fifty in fact – carry a bacterium called *Helicobacter pylori* in our stomachs. This bug can be a contributing factor in acid indigestion symptoms, so it needs to be eradicated. This is done by taking two different high-strength antibiotics and a high-dose acid blocker for one week. We call this triple therapy. Although it sounds drastic, for many people banishing this bug serves not only to sort symptoms, but also to prevent ulcers and in some cases stomach cancer.

Referral

If your symptoms are unusual or severe, you are losing weight, you are over fifty, your iron is low or your pain is constant, you should seek advice from a gastroenterologist. Such a referral generally includes having a telescope passed through the oesophagus into the stomach and on into the duodenum. It's the gold standard in diagnosing ulcers. If you are found to have an ulcer, medication is so good nowadays that surgery is rarely needed as pills can generally heal it. However, ignore an ulcer at your peril as it can perforate and you could bleed to death.

Your role

Use your common sense and avoid triggers like white wine, curries and eating late at night. Another pitfall is drinking fluids late at night – this aggravates night-time acid. Tight clothing such as corsets, stooping and lying totally flat in bed at night (elevate the bed head) all make symptoms worse.

Tip *Coughing during the night can be a sign of acid reflux.*

GALLSTONES

WHERE IS YOUR GALLBLADDER?

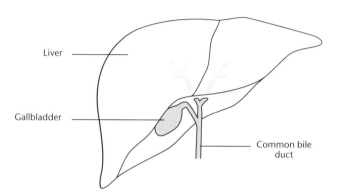

Liver

Gallbladder

Common bile
duct

Who gets them?

Most medical students could reel off the risk factors for gallstones – Female, Fair, Fat, Forty and Fertile. Very often there is a family history too. Bizarrely, although gallstones are common in those who are overweight, you can also get them if you lose weight rapidly. Also, people with diabetes or liver disease are also prone to them.

What are they?

Have a look at the diagram above – there is a little bag-shaped organ on the right hand side of the body that sits just below the liver. This is called the gallbladder, and it stores a green liquid called bile which the liver makes to break down fats and other substances. If you have ever had a bad vomiting bug and ended up bringing up putrid green stuff, that's bile.

When you eat, bile is released from your gallbladder into your gut through the bile duct. Bile contains cholesterol, bile salts and waste products, and gallstones form when these solidify or harden.

How would I know I had them?

You may not. Gallstones are very common and you often don't know you have them until you have an 'attack'. One in ten people will develop gallstones, but there is no need to worry about this as gallstones that don't cause symptoms don't need treatment.

Mischievous gallstones can irritate the gallbladder or get stuck in the bile duct. When a stone gets stuck in the bile duct, you get an attack of colic. This is the description given to any type of pain with peaks and troughs, like labour pains. Biliary colic often presents with pain in the belly under the right rib cage, with sweating, fever, restlessness and sometimes even jaundice (yellowing of the skin).

Gallstones can't be diagnosed by means of an X-ray. Instead you need an ultrasound scan, similar to the scans done during pregnancy. If you have had attacks of pain after fatty meals and you fit the identikit of the gallstone lady, talk to your doctor about having a test. Confirming gallstones doesn't mean you have to have an operation, but it does mean you will have a explanation for your pain and can help to prevent further episodes or at least deal with them when they occur.

Treatment If you discover you have gallstones but they aren't giving you grief, leave them alone.

Recurrent attacks of gallstones require action You can live without your gallbladder. Using a telescope with a set of tweezers and cutting instruments, it can be whipped out of your belly in less than ninety minutes. This leaves only minor scarring and is done under general anaesthetic – we call this a laparoscopic cholecystectomy.

Fewer than 10 per cent of people will need open cholecystectomy, which requires a 12–20cm (5–8in) incision across the abdomen. This requires a longer stay in hospital, and you are more prone to complications such as infection. It is usually resorted to in very obese patients as it can be impossible to undertake keyhole surgery due to their bulk.

Stones can also be removed from the bile duct by a procedure called ERCP. They can also be dissolved by ingesting medicines, but this can take months or years.

Watch out
▮ *Women are twice as likely as men to suffer from gallstones.*
▮ *An attack of gallstones often comes on after eating a fatty meal.*
▮ *If your mum had gallstones, you are highly likely to suffer too. Ditch the fat, don't crash diet and keep your cholesterol in check.*

Skin

12

Respect the skin as it's the largest organ in the body and you wear it every day of the week. Read on to find out what can go wrong and where to find help.

ACNE

Eighty per cent of us get acne at some point, and when we do we put one hundred per cent into getting rid of it! Although we think of acne as teenage trouble, spots start to sprout in 5 per cent of women aged between twenty-five and forty. It is due to an excess of a substance called sebum. Even the name sounds greasy. Our pilosebaceous glands are effectively what lie behind the pores in our skin. They are attached to the hair follicles and produce oil – the sebum.

So why does acne just flare up?

As a rule of thumb, all 'spots' are acne and all acne lesions are 'spots'. There isn't a specific definition of a spot. Blackheads, whiteheads, papules and pustules – most of us have been there. But why? Excessive secretion of sebum seems to be the problem. Our system is very sensitive to circulating levels of the hormone testosterone, and this results in an excessive production of sebum. And before you start worrying about having testosterone, all women have a small amount – it's quite normal. In addition to the excess grease, we also get irregular shedding of the skin cells so the follicle becomes blocked. The grease inside then allows bacteria called *Propionibacterium acnes*, natural skin inhabitants, to multiply. On the outside, the follicle wall bulges and produces a whitehead. If the plug opens to the surface, the plug appears as a blackhead. The technical term for blackheads and whiteheads is comedones.

EXCESSIVE SEBUM IN THE HAIR FOLICLE

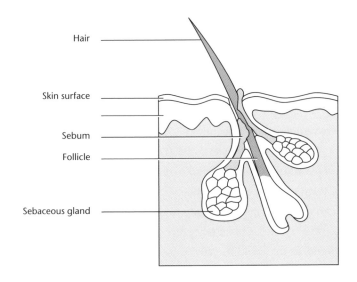

Hair

Skin surface

Sebum

Follicle

Sebaceous gland

205

Surely in the twenty-first century there is a cure?

No, acne can't be cured. However, that doesn't mean it can't be treated. The simplest approach is buying a tube of benzoyl peroxide from your pharmacist. Isn't peroxide what you use to clean the toilet? No, this treatment is very clever and is the first line of acne attack. It has antibacterial action against Propionibacterium acnes and also helps to remove the dead skin cells blocking the follicle. It is smart, cheap and available in different formulations.

What's available on prescription?

The doctor will often prescribe topical treatments to be applied. These might include an antibiotic, which can be combined with benzoyl peroxide for extra action against the bacteria as well as to get rid of excess skin cells. Retinoids work directly on the skin cells and loosen them, preventing them blocking the follicles. Azelaic acid preparations increase cell turnover and are antibacterial too. There are, however, two issues with all treatments you apply. First, they may initially irritate your skin. If so, simply reduce the frequency of application and use only a pea-sized amount to cover the face. Second, it could be four to twelve weeks before anything happens, so you need to persist.

Follow-up

Be honest when you go back to your doctor. Tell them if you didn't like your treatment, didn't use it or didn't see any benefit. Doctors aren't stupid – we know some of you don't even take the prescription to the pharmacist! It may just be that it isn't working for you. Equally, don't continue to collect repeat prescriptions if nothing's clearing.

Pills

We ladies are lucky as we have the oral contraceptive pill as a treatment option. The one containing cyproterone acetate and ethinylestradiol (Dianette, Diane) works by reducing the amount of male hormone circulating so decreases its effect on sebum production. This is the ideal choice in those needing contraception and those with polycystic ovary syndrome. Other pills containing newer progesterones such as drospirenone (Yasmin) also work well. Conversely, steer clear of pills containing norethisterone (norethindrone) as this could be causing your spots.

Antibiotics

The 'anti-bugs' get very bad press – the acne bacteria are building up resistance so they are becoming less effective. In the first instance, you will be offered a tetracycline antibiotic, erythromycin or clindamycin. It makes sense to combine these with other treatments to boost their effects. So use a benzoyl peroxide gel or a retinoid as well.

What if nothing works?

If the topical and oral medications aren't effective, your next port of call is a dermatologist, who will discuss isotretinoin (Roaccutane, Accutane, Oratane) with you. This drug reduces sebum production and also loosens skin cells, so there is less grease and less pore blockage. It's potent stuff, so before you take it you will be talked through its side-effects. Because it is broken down in your liver and can have an effect on your blood, you need a blood test first. You also need a pregnancy test because isotretinoin directly affects the unborn baby. Dermatologists will require all women to take oral contraception while on isotretinoin, as well as to have a pregnancy test every month.

So although this treatment is very effective, it is not simply a question of popping a pill. It requires a lot of input from you. Booze binges are out because of its liver effects, as are sun beds, waxes and blood donation. Some people can feel down in the dumps while taking it, so it is important to talk through all aspects of your life with the doctor before contemplating it.

Acne scars

Beware the picking and popping of spots. Acne scars tend to be worse on darker skin. If you are left with a reminder of your adolescent acne, laser treatment might be an option, but every scar is different.

Tip

Beware the bleach in benzoyl peroxide as it stains clothes.

Use water-based non-comedogenic cosmetics as they are less spot-stimulating.

Myths

Acne is caused by dirty skin, chips, chocolate and stress. No. If you find a food that drives your acne crazy, then of course kick it, but you don't have to avoid all your vices.

You must scrub your skin clean. No, as this can actually make acne worse. Wash twice a day with a mild soap.

THE ECZEMA FAMILY

The word eczema comes from the Greek meaning to boil. Just as an irritating person can make your blood boil, external and internal irritants make your skin 'boil' and give you eczema. About one in twelve adults have it, and as many as one in five kids. Although it tends to burn itself out before they're in double figures, it can crop up again in adulthood.

Classically, the skin looks dry, red and scaly and tends to be very irritated. Eczema crops up in the bends of the elbow and knees, at the wrists and on the back of the neck. Wherever there is skin, there can potentially be eczema. We tend to use the words eczema and dermatitis interchangeably to refer to any itchy, irritant skin rash.

Can you catch eczema?

You can't catch eczema or physically pass it on. It is, however, inherited through your genes, so if a family member has eczema, asthma or hay fever, you are more likely to suffer. We call these three conditions the atopic triad and the associated skin condition atopic eczema. It is thought to be due to an exaggerated immune response. If you have an atopic condition, your child has a one in four chance of some form of atopic disease. If both you and your partner are atopic, your child has a one in two chance.

Are you born with eczema or can you develop it?

As well as being born with the tendency to suffer from eczema, it is possible to develop it from exposure to substances such as chemicals in the workplace – we call this contact dermatitis. Seborrhoeic eczema is the term given to the type of eczema that gives rise to cradle cap in babies and dandruff in adults. Eczema can also arise where the circulation is poor, such as over varicose veins. And an itchy patch of skin can often develop into eczema due to chronic scratching – we call this neurodermatitis. Finally, there is pompholyx eczema, which typically affects the hands and feet, with blisters, itching and a burning sensation. This type is twice as common in women as men.

Is there a test for eczema?

There's no specific test, and in mild cases none is warranted as the diagnosis is easy to establish based on talking to the individual and looking at the skin. If there's any doubt, you may be referred for a skin biopsy, in which a tiny piece of skin is analysed under the microscope. If a chemical irritation or allergy is suspected, you may also have blood or patch tests. Patch tests involve putting chemicals onto the skin and seeing how it reacts after forty-eight hours.

What flares eczema up?

Eczema is affected by how you feel, so if you are stressed, run down or ill, your symptoms may worsen. Heat, sweat, extreme cold or central heating can also flare it, as can toxins such as alcohol. Anything that dries the skin may cause a flare, which is why eczema seems to be worse during the winter. Chemicals in washing powders, wool, pollen, pets, you name it, the household is a hazard! In addition, 30 per cent of women experience a flare of their eczema premenstrually, and 50 per cent in pregnancy.

What are the complications?

Eczema can become infected. We all carry bugs on our skin, and one in particular, *Staphylococcus aureus,* can cause eczema to become infected if present in large amounts. This can result in very inflamed skin that is crusty, weeping and very itchy. Persistent itching and scratching can damage the skin, resulting in thickening and discoloration. And persistent irritation and scratching at night can really disturb sleep. Because patients with eczema wear their condition, it can have a significant psychological impact, too.

Can it be cured?

No, your potential to have eczema will go to the grave with you. However, with a good skin management plan, you should be able to keep it under control. Work with your doctor or practice nurse in deciding which treatment is best for you and which you are likely to use.

Watering our dry skin

Moisturising the skin is a key component of any plan. Often, however, patients foolishly use layer upon layer of moisturiser, which has the effect of trapping heat as well as moisture so makes the skin feel hot, irritated and itchy. Moisturiser should be put on like fake tan – simply a shimmer to give the skin a shine, and no need to rub it in. The other issue is that many of the moisturisers we prescribe are smelly, sticky and offensive! These creams can make driving difficult, ruin our clothes and create blobs all over our business documents. As such, it is vital to find an effective moisturiser that is a treat rather than a trial to use. Then apply this frequently, thinly and gently.

Don't want steroids?

There are two types of patient: ones who never use steroids and ones who overuse them. The golden rules are not to use other people's steroid creams, and when using your own to stick to the designated areas and dosage. Less is not more in the context of topical steroids – steroid side-effects occur because of inappropriate usage.

We measure steroid dosage in fingertip units. One fingertip unit is the amount that comes out of a tube squeezed along an adult's fingertip. It's enough to treat an area twice the size of the flat of your hand with your fingers closed up. So treating an entire leg and foot requires eight fingertip units. Got it? See the diagram to make sense of it.

There are numerous side-effects of steroids but if steroids are used as prescribed, they are generally safe. They can, however, cause thinning of the skin, stretch marks, bruising and colour changes. On the face, they can lead to acne and spider veins. It is exceptionally rare though to see side-effects from steroids being absorbed into the bloodstream.

RECOMMENDED UNITS OF CREAM TO APPLY

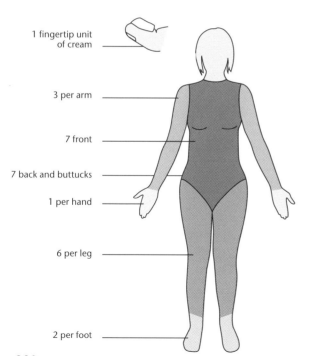

1 fingertip unit of cream

3 per arm

7 front

7 back and buttucks

1 per hand

6 per leg

2 per foot

Getting the best out of your medicine

Ideally, you want to get the maximum effect from the minimum steroid application. As it works best on well-hydrated skin, moisturise your skin regularly. Try to let the moisturiser sink in for about fifteen minutes first. Then apply your steroid and if possible do nothing for fifteen minutes. Even better, apply clingfilm over the area and this will help to sweat the treatment into the skin.

When your eczema starts to settle, count how may days it took to get to the 'looking good' point and then keep using the treatment for 50 per cent of that time. This is because although the skin looks fine on the surface, there is still activity underneath and stopping abruptly will result in a flare –you'll end up at square one again.

Are there alternatives to steroids?

Yes, creams containing tacrolimus and protacrolimus can be used when other creams fail, but they can't be used on a continuous basis. They work by affecting the skin's immune response and were developed from a medicine used to prevent transplant patients rejecting organs. They serve to control moderate to severe eczema and also decrease the itch. Their safety when used over long periods of time has, however, not yet been established.

What about pills?

Oral steroids are reserved for severe flare-ups of eczema and are not the mainstay of treatment due to their side-effects. Antibiotic tablets are necessary if you experience an infection, and your doctor may also prescribe an antibiotic ointment. Serious eczema may require treatment with drugs that suppress the immune response, but these are only available from a dermatologist as they require strict monitoring. Antihistamines can be helpful to break the itch–scratch cycle.

Tip *Always opt for an ointment above a cream. Ointments contain no alcohol so do not irritate the skin and do not evaporate easily. They are ideal for dry, cracked skin.*

Self-help

Scratch any part of your skin for long enough and it will start to look like eczema. So establish your most scratchy times of the day and try to break the habit. Keep your hands busy, and if you insist on having a go at your skin, try to pinch or press the area rather than scratching it. Beware the pitfalls of excessively rubbing the skin, for example when applying treatments or drying yourself after a shower. Save the planet and your skin by not taking a bath and by spending only five minutes in a tepid shower; this also prevents the drying effects of hot hard water.

Tips

▌ *Don't suffer in silence. If your eczema is getting on top of you, do something about it. Don't pretend to the doctor that you are using your creams if you are not – be honest and explain why. As you can develop a sensitivity to ingredients in the creams, go back to your doctor if a treatment seems to be making things worse. And talk to your doctor about how you are and not just how your eczema is. Also, don't stay on the same treatment for years – arrange a twice-yearly review to check out new options.*

▌ *Control your eczema by means of a good treatment plan, otherwise it will control you.*

▌ *Never stop moisturising as this is the key to flake-free skin, and use steroids sensibly. Cut your fingernails short as they are the enemy in terms of night-time scratching.*

HAND DERMATITIS

The terms eczema and dermatitis are used interchangeably. I tend to reserve 'eczema' for the atopic variety – the type associated with asthma and hay fever that is common in children. We can then call all the others dermatitis.

What might my hands look like?

They will be dry, cracked, flaky, red and sore. They may even bleed, and they will be irritated by even simple things such as soap.

With all the different types of dermatitis mostly looking the same, what's the solution to diagnosis?

Diagnosis is actually fairly straightforward and is based on the site and trigger factors. For contact irritant dermatitis, we'll look to see if we can find an offending substance or substances, such as harsh chemicals. Hairdressers, for example, should beware the combination of latex gloves, hair dye and water.

In allergic contact dermatitis, your immune system reacts to a substance because it signals it's allergic to it. Nickel is a common one, so when working at a change counter you might see patches on your hands in response to handling coins. Broadly speaking, the irritant-type dermatitis is due to overexposure and the other type to allergy. Dry skin can give rise to dermatitis and is more common in the menopause. Anything that causes dryness can result in dermatitis, for example cold weather or excessive hand washing, as seen with healthcare workers.

A helping hand

If you suffer from hand dermatitis, always carry a soap substitute, such as aqueous cream, with you – soaps and hand sanitisers in public places contain harsh detergents. If you are doing the washing up, wear cotton gloves under rubber ones (the cotton gloves will stop you sweating, which will cause skin irritation). Also wear gloves to avoid direct contact when preparing foods such as onions, lemons, garlic and fruit. And do the same when you are using cleaning products in the home.

Ten per cent of women have some degree of hand dermatitis, a typical trigger being a newborn baby as this brings with it regular hand washing. Make sure too that you take your rings off before hand-washing or wet work, and pat your hands dry.

Tip *Wear vinyl gloves when washing your hair to protect your hands.*

Still can't handle it?

See your doctor as it may be worth having some specialist tests to check for specific allergies. These patch tests will identify the irritants you may be coming into contact with. Small amounts of possible culprits are applied to your skin and the reaction is checked by a specialist forty-eight hours later. It is always worth asking your doctor to do blood tests for allergy levels and to rule out other underlying problems.

FLAKY SCALP

A flaky scalp is incredibly common, and the signs can vary from dandruff to seborrhoeic dermatitis. Dandruff is simply snowflakes falling from the scalp, whereas seborrhoeic dermatitis leads to skin that is flaky and inflamed, making it red, itchy and sore.

How do I know which it is?

Seborrhoeic dermatitis is usually severe dandruff and both embarrasses and irritates you. You will often scratch your scalp so much that it bleeds. Unfortunately, simple antidandruff shampoos don't do the trick. The flake seems to migrate onto the eyebrows, eyelashes and face, giving you flaky red skin on your cheeks and between your brows.

What's the problem?

We all have yeast living on our skin, and it is thought that an overgrowth of a yeast called *Malassezia* causes the problem. Hormones play a role too as the seborrhoeic dermatitis of adults is the same as the cradle cap of babies when they are born (it's even treated the same way) – yet the condition has disappeared in childhood only to return with the hormonal surge of adolescence. Stress, alcohol, low immunity (e.g. HIV) and neurological problems such as Parkinson's disease can also trigger it.

Fix the flake!

▊ Avoid triggers such as stress and alcohol as they make it worse.

▊ Use a shampoo with ketoconazole in to kill off the yeast.

▊ You may need topical steroid gels or mousses to damp down the inflammation, and preparations with salicylic acid in to help descale the scalp.

▊ Recurrent attacks of this condition might signal that your immune system is poor, so you should talk to your doctor about having some blood tests.

Because ketoconazole shampoo is sold over the counter in many countries and is used a lot, some yeasts are now resistant to it – if the shampoo isn't helping, ask your doctor for something on prescription.

Is the diagnosis right?

Another cause for flaky scalp is psoriasis. This should be considered if the flakiness is very severe, you have psoriasis elsewhere on your body or it runs in your family. Don't forget to mention any problems with your nails or joints as even if you don't think you have psoriasis, these could seal the deal for a doctor's diagnosis of psoriasis. And rather than just talking to the doctor about your scalp, make sure they get up close and personal with it to get a picture of its severity.

Tip ▊ *Beware the flaky scalp – ignore it and your face may pay the price, so break out the anti-yeast shampoo.*

ALLERGY AND URTICARIA

You know when you come into contact with an obnoxious man, your body signals that you want to repel him! Well, when your body comes into contact with a protein that it considers noxious and mounts an immune response against it, that's an allergy. About one in every three people suffer from an allergy, and it's on the increase. It's possible to be allergic to sperm, water, even sunlight; 15 per cent of urticaria is caused by cold, heat, light or exercise, so even a simple shower may induce it. Around 90 per cent of food allergies are due to nuts, fish, shellfish, eggs, meat, wheat and soy.

What about food allergies?

Food allergies occur either immediately on ingesting the food or a couple of hours later during digestion. There will generally be itching, a nettle rash, stomach discomfort, diarrhoea or vomiting. Occasionally, there will be an asthmatic attack or a full-blown anaphylactic reaction in which the throat closes up or the person even collapses. Nuts, fish, wheat, eggs, soy and kiwi are common culprits. Levels of the antibody IgE rise in the bloodstream as this substance flies into action at the threat of, for example, a peanut.

Is it possible to have food allergies and not have any symptoms?

You'll often have a food intolerance, which means you don't mount a full allergic reaction but your body signals it isn't happy. This will never result in a full-blown allergy attack.

What's oral allergy syndrome?

In this strange situation, if you are a hay fever sufferer, certain fresh fruits, vegetables and nuts trigger an allergic reaction as soon as they are eaten. This is because there are similarities between the proteins in the pollen and those in the particular foods, and your body creates a crossreaction. There are many weird interconnections, so if you are allergic to grass pollen, you may react to tomato and kiwi fruit. Or if silver birch makes you sneeze, you might find raw carrots and celery hard to swallow. Your mouth will tingle and itch, and your throat may start to swell. But if you suffer from this, cooking the foods breaks up the proteins so you no longer react.

Are hives and urticaria the same thing?

Yes, they're red, raised areas of skin that tend to itch. They are caused by histamine – the substance that causes the skin reaction to nettle stings. Hives can last for minutes or hours – they're acute if episodes occur over a period of six weeks or less, and chronic when attacks come back periodically, sometimes for years. Often, we never discover what is causing it. Middle-aged women tend to suffer from chronic hives more than men. Having said that, 20 per cent of us will be struck at some point.

How can I calm the reaction down?

If you are experiencing difficulty breathing or swallowing, call the emergency services. An antihistamine is the first choice for home treatment. With a severe case, the doctor may prescribe a course of steroids or advise two different antihistamines to be taken simultaneously. Be cautious with driving when you are on antihistamines, and don't drink alcohol.

Why can't the doctor work out what's wrong?

Chronic urticaria tends to be your body reacting to yourself and no cause is established. You can have numerous tests to rule things out, but frustratingly they're often unable to rule a cause in. However, you should try to avoid stress, extreme changes in temperature, aspirin, red wine and foodstuffs with tartrazine in. Tomatoes, strawberries and strong cheese can potentially aggravate the condition, so ban these too. Weirdly, it tends to resolve spontaneously over a period of months, although the urticaria may linger for years.

Tips   *If in any doubt about your hives, ask your doctor about infections, lupus and thyroid problems.*

Try a non-drowsy antihistamine by day and a sedating one by night. Switch antihistamines periodically if their effectiveness seems to dwindle.

PSORIASIS

What is psoriasis?

Many people confuse eczema with psoriasis. Psoriasis occurs when the process of shedding skin cells takes forty-eight hours to a week rather than the standard three to four weeks. So instead of the leaves coming off the trees in autumn and being replaced in spring, it's akin to having 'fall' every month. It's not a new condition – signs of it have even been seen in Egyptian mummies.

What does it look like?

The vast number of skin cells shed tend to accumulate on the skin surface in the form of raised patches with redness beneath and silvery scales on top. If you scratch these, they can bleed easily. They tend to crop up on the backs of the elbows and the front of the knees – the opposite of eczema – as well as on the lower back. Psoriasis can also occur on the scalp, giving rise to scaling and itchy plaques that often bleed. It also occasionally occurs in the nails, making them crumbly and resulting in tiny pits in the nail bed.

How do I catch it?

It's not a question of catching it as it's not an infection or infestation. About 2 to 3 per cent of the world's population are affected. It's most common in Western Europe and Scandinavia, but rare in people from West Africa. In 30 per cent of cases there is a family history.

The key time for it to appear is between ten and forty years of age, often triggered by puberty – only 10 per cent of adults with psoriasis had the condition before the age of ten. It is thought to be caused by a combination of factors, namely our genes, our environment and our immune system.

What starts it off?

Sometimes nothing, but stress, either mental or physical, often serves as a trigger, as can something as simple as a sore throat or pregnancy.

How do I get rid of it?

Sadly, there is no cure, and anyone who tells you different is lying. But treatments can help with the symptoms. Unfortunately, over one hundred million people worldwide have psoriasis, yet only half of these receive proper treatment.

The cornerstone of psoriasis treatment is skin moisturisation, before you even begin to apply prescription preparations. After that, a mixture of the drug calcipotriol (calcipotriene) and a steroid in an ointment is an excellent choice if psoriasis is affecting 30 per cent of your skin. Steroids on their own can also be used, and tend to soothe psoriasis on the backs of the joints. Another product called dithranol (anthralin) can be applied, but it is very irritating and should only be applied for less than sixty minutes. Sadly, ladies, it also stains the skin brown.

Cold tar preparations are still also used; they can be messy but, for reasons unknown to science, they tend to work well and are excellent for scalp psoriasis. They do, however, stink!

If you have bad nail psoriasis or severe psoriasis all over the body, standard creams and lotions often don't work, so you may be referred to a dermatologist for tablets. These drugs target your immune system and cell division, so blood tests must be done first and you must follow a rigid management plan. They are not compatible with pregnancy, so any plans you have of becoming pregnant will have to be shelved and you will have to take the oral contraceptive pill before you can start treatment.

Sunlight Anecdotally, sunlight helps psoriasis, so a sunny holiday is the best medicine. Dermatology clinics also offer light treatment (called PUVA) to selected patients. Great care, however, has to be taken to avoid burning the skin, and there is an increased risk of skin cancer. In addition, light treatment is time-consuming, resulting in weekly visits to the outpatient clinic for many months.

The Dead Sea This lies between Israel and Jordan and, at 400m below sea level, is the lowest point on earth. Its salt content is ten times that of the ordinary sea. Its waters are rich in salts and minerals, and as a result of the high content of these, you simply cannot sink. It also has incredibly beneficial effects on psoriasis.

Wearing your condition

You wear psoriasis for all to see, and it can have a huge psychological impact on those who have it. Ironically, it used to be mistaken for leprosy until it was finally given the name psoriasis in 1841. An estimated 10 per cent of women with severe psoriasis have suicidal thoughts. Many women do not embark on sexual relationships because of it and feel that it holds them back both personally and professionally. Psoriasis isn't simply skin deep, and although there isn't a cure, keep knocking on the doctor's door for help.

Tips

If you have really bad dandruff, see the doctor. This might be mild psoriasis and could be treated with medicated shampoos and ointments.

Beware party time as the toxins you take in will tip your skin into overproduction and stress your psoriasis.

Crumbly nails with little pits in them … it may not be a fungus. See the doctor as this could be psoriasis.

KERATOSIS PILARIS

This condition can be summed up in two words – chicken skin! Yes, that's what it looks like, ladies, and we're not terribly fond of having it.

Where does it occur, and what is it?

It's usually found on the back of the upper arms, the thighs or the buttocks, and occasionally on the cheeks. It's a result of keratin blocking the hair follicles instead of being exfoliated. This makes the pores widen so the plug looks bigger. The condition appears like goose bumps that can sometimes become red and inflamed. It can look like acne and often feels like sandpaper.

Who gets it?

It is more common in ladies, and about 40 per cent of women suffer. It generally starts in puberty, although it can occur at any age. It is more commonly seen in people with very dry skin or who have eczema, asthma or hay fever. And it generally runs in families.

Can I cure it?

Unfortunately no, but it often resolves spontaneously. If it doesn't clear up, don't worry as it hasn't got any long-term consequences, but there are things you can do to help it. Keep your skin well hydrated, and make sure you exfoliate weekly. Don't be tempted to scratch it as this can cause depigmentation or overpigmentation of the skin and leave you with marks. Urea cream is a good moisturiser, or you can try ones with alphahydroxyacids in. Some treatments for acne, such as creams with retinol A or azelaic acid, have been used. However, these are only available on prescription, and using them is very much a case of trial and error. Laser treatment tends to reduce the redness but not the bumpiness. Finally, fake tan serves as a good method of camouflage. Remember, you aren't alone – check everyone else's arms and you'll find that four out of ten of your friends have a bit of chicken skin too.

SCARS

Scarring is a necessary evil – it occurs as a result of how our skin heals after an injury or operation. Scars can, however, be unsightly and distressing.

How do you scar?

There is a complex relationship between wound healing and the laying down of collagen and connective tissues in the skin. Wounds from accidents are more likely to give irregular scars as the cut itself will be irregular. But straight surgical wounds can also scar. And some people are more prone to what is called hypertrophic – keloid – scarring. This can sometimes be seen in the aftermath of acne, an operation or an accident.

What do these keloids look like?

They tend to be thick, red, raised scars that stand out from the skin. The most common sites are the chest, back and face. Afro-Caribbean skin is most likely to suffer, and there is also often a genetic predisposition. The problem is that you cannot really cut a keloid scar out because you are then likely to produce another scar. Caught between a rock and a hard place? Not necessarily. Keloids can be treated with steroid creams in an effort to minimise the redness and flatten the scar. It is also possible to inject them with steroids if the creams don't work. A type of steroid tape available on prescription can be applied over the keloid. And scarring can be treated with lasers, which help to flatten and de-pigment it.

Words of advice – if you have acne, don't pick at it

You run the risk of scarring, even keloid, which may be with you for years after your acne has gone. Don't have benign skin moles and lumps removed just because you don't like the look of them. The scar produced may end up being more obvious than the original lesion. Vitamin E cream is good for postoperative scars, and severe scars can be helped with silicone gel. Protect your scar from the sun as it is more likely to burn. Remember that there is no surgery without scarring.

SHAVING BUMPS

This may sound like it's one for the guys, but the girls have problems with it too.

What happens?

When the hair grows back after shaving, it can grow inwards. This can result in inflammation and redness around and in the hair follicle. The follicle can also sometimes become infected as a result, and we call this folliculitis.

Does that mean I shouldn't shave?

No, it doesn't, but when you are choosing a razor, don't go for a double blade as this shaves too close to your skin and you are far more likely to get 'razor bumps', as the lads call them. Remember that curly hair is far more likely to grow inwards after shaving, so this is a particular problem with pubic hair.

What can I do to prevent it?

Prepare your skin before you pounce by moisturising it, and use a shaving gel or foam during shaving. Remember to shave in the direction of the hair rather than against it. And exfoliate the area with a product containing glycolic acid the night before as it is then far less likely to become inflamed. Using an antiseptic like tea tree oil before and afterwards can also be of benefit.

The golden rules of razors

Remember to throw your razor out after a few weeks if it's disposable, otherwise it will harbour germs that can cause the hair follicles to become infected. If you have an electric shaver, make sure you cleanse it regularly with an antibacterial agent as again it can harbour bugs and give rise to infections. If you do get these bugs into your skin, you can develop folliculitis; this often requires a course of antibiotics to clear it.

And finally, the golden rule of razors dictates that you should never, ever, ever use your partner's razor to shave your armpits or your downstairs bits. You are highly likely to transfer bacteria from their razor to your skin and set the chain in motion for infection and inflammation.

WARTS

Nobody wants to have a wart! They generally tend to crop up on the hands and the feet – when they're in the latter site, we refer to them as verrucas. At this moment in time, as many as one in ten of the population will have a wart lurking somewhere. Left alone, they tend to disappear in a couple of years in most cases. They can run in families, often because they spread from one source to another.

How do I get rid of them?

You can buy salicylic acid at the pharmacist and apply it every night for at least eight weeks. It is important to pare down the dead skin around the wart – you can do this with a nail file, and the treatment pack often comes with one. It is also a good idea to leave the wart covered with a sticking plaster after applying the salicylic acid. Because salicylic acid is, as the name says, an acid, try not to get it on the unaffected skin as it will irritate it. Remember that you won't notice any difference for at least two weeks, and it often takes three months before things start to clear up.

Give it frost bite If home measures do not work, you can have the wart frozen with liquid nitrogen. Just as the salicylic acid burns the wart with acid, so freezing therapy kills it with extreme cold. The procedure can be uncomfortable, and you can occasionally get blisters afterwards. This is not, however, a one-hit wonder, and it often requires three or four treatments several weeks apart.

Immunotherapy Troublesome warts and verrucas can be treated with immunotherapy in specialist centres. This involves applying a caustic chemical to the skin that stimulates a reaction within the skin. This in turn triggers an immune response that kills off the wart virus.

What's the alternative? Some research suggests that electrical tape applied for six days out of seven can help to get rid of warts and verrucas if used for a period of eight weeks. One thing is for sure, it is unlikely to do any harm, but the jury is still out on the scientific evidence behind its success.

When a wart has another meaning

If you suddenly develop warts out of the blue, see your doctor for a blood test as this could be the first sign of a problem with your immune system. And beware the man with a facial wart as this could be sexually transmitted.

FUNGAL INFECTION

Lots of us are infected with fungus! It sounds horrid, but luckily the diagnosis and treatment are straightforward.

Who gets fungal infections?

Anyone really, but these infections are more common after taking antibiotics or steroid tablets or if you have diabetes, you are obese or your immunity is low, for example with cancer or HIV.

What makes the fungus grow?

Think of how mould grows in a cupboard – well, it's exactly the same. Skin that is moist, humid and kept in darkness is an ideal breeding ground. So think sweating, or wetness after showering – that's fungus party time.

How does it spread?

Fungus spreads by direct contact with someone's skin or with areas that have been used by people with fungus. That's why the gym is a great source of it. Our friendly pets can also transmit fungus.

What should I look out for?

Check out the fungus menu below and see what's what.

Athlete's foot This is probably the most common fungus and you may inadvertently pass it on to a friend or partner as your skin sheds contaminated skin particles. It is easily treated with cream bought from the pharmacy.

Fungal nails These look thick and yellow and tend to crumble when cut. This condition usually affects the toenails, and there is often co-existing athlete's foot between the toes – it's this that spreads and causes the nasty nails. The nails can be treated with medicated nail lacquer, but you often need a three to six month course of pills. It is imperative that you have liver tests before you take these tablets as they are broken down in the liver.

Groin itch This tends to be one for the boys, but the girls get it too. Here fungus causes an itchy, flaky, red rash in the groins. This is very common in sweaty groins, so beware those tight lycras in the gym. We tell men, socks before jocks ... women with athlete's foot should do the same.

Ringworm Meet the all-over body fungus. You can spot this as it is classically ring-shaped – hence the name – and the centre tends to be clear. You can catch it from cats, dogs or cattle and spread it to all the family.

Tip *An innocent patch of eczema may actually be fungus. Consider this if it is not clearing.*

Pitfall *Never assume that nails are infected with fungus – always ask your doctor to send clippings to the lab to confirm the diagnosis. Psoriasis of the nails can look like fungus so you may be treating the wrong thing.*

MELASMA

Melasma – the pregnancy mask

Have you ever wondered why a pregnant pal seems to be wearing smudged make-up? That's melasma, in which you get excessive brown pigment appearing on the cheeks, nose, forehead, chin or upper lip. It's often called the mask of pregnancy.

Can anyone else get melasma?

Ninety per cent of those who suffer are women, and melasma runs in families. Those with darker skin who live in warmer climes seem to be more susceptible. It's often seen with pregnancy, hormone replacement therapy and the oral contraceptive pill. When hormone status reverts to normal, i.e. you stop the pill or deliver your baby, the pigment often, but not always, starts to fade. The sun acts as an incubator and 'brings out' the pigment patches. Sufferers find this very distressing as it looks like a stain on the face or even a moustache.

What do you do?

First and foremost, talk to your doctor. If you are pregnant, you can be offered azelaic acid, an acne treatment safe in pregnancy that can help to make it fade. If you are on the oral contraceptive pill, switch to an alternative form of contraception. If that's not practical, change pills. Bleaching creams containing hydroquinone 4 per cent usually are available on prescription. Other treatments used are retinoid creams, again an acne treatment. These work to bleach what is already there and prevent further activity in the pigment cells. Dermabrasion and chemical peels can work to remove surface pigmentation. It is vital to have this done by a skilled professional as it could give rise to further patches of pigmentation or depigmentation. The use of lasers is still evolving, but intense pulsed-light lasers seem promising. And above all, it's a case of sun block, sun block, sun block! Use a preparation with both zinc oxide and titanium dioxide with an SPF of 30. It's vital you use this every day of the year as it prevents new pigment forming as well as preventing reoccurrence if you have already achieved a cure.

Tip ▌ *Avoid scented toiletries and cosmetics as they can make you even more light-sensitive.*

STRETCH MARKS

We simply hate these! Rapid stretching of the skin causes a break or overstretch in the layer called the dermis, which contains the collagen and elastin that give the skin its elastic quality. It initially looks red as what you are seeing is a break in the skin, the redness being the blood vessels showing through. After a while, these vessels contract down so the marks appear white. They fade but never truly disappear, and occur most commonly on the abdomen, upper arms, breasts and thighs.

Who gets them?

Stretch marks are incredibly common in puberty due to hormones and the growth spurt. The same is true of pregnancy. Any rapid weight loss or gain can cause them, so beware you permarexics – permanently on a diet, raisins this week, eggs the next. Stretch marks are also sometimes seen in people who take steroids, for example for body-building or medical reasons, and in those who produce too much steroid because of an adrenal gland problem. Topical steroids shouldn't give you stretch marks if used correctly. A classic pitfall area is the groin, where the skin is thin.

So how do I get rid of them?

Unfortunately, you can't. But you can try not to get any more. In the early stages, laser can be used on the red marks to fade them more quickly, but the older the mark, the less likely it is to help. A post-pregnancy belly with stretch marks and excess fat could be helped by abdominoplasty – a tummy tuck – but that's a big operation for a belly that only goes on display two weeks a year in Majorca. Think very seriously first.

Do creams work? All manner of things – collagen creams, oils, cocoa products – say they'll rid you of stretch marks. The testimonials outweigh the scientific evidence, but if you a find a product that's safe and seems to work, go for it!

Tips

Don't abuse or overuse steroids.

Don't yo-yo diet.

Do consider camouflage make-up.

MOLES

One episode of sunburn before the age of twenty doubles your lifetime risk of skin cancer. Yes, that's fact. But although we are all sun-smart, are we skin aware … would you know what to spot?

Skin cancer is on the up and is one of the most common cancers in the UK today: the incidence of melanoma has quadrupled since I was born in the 1970s. It is mostly caused by exposure to ultraviolet light, either real from the sun or artificial from sunbeds. More women develop it than men, and it's often ladies' legs that are involved.

What should I be looking for?

Know your moles. A safe mole should:

- Be symmetrical
- Have regular edges
- Have an even colour
- Be smaller than the head of a pencil.

And know the ABCD rule. Look for: Asymmetry, Borders, Colour and Diameter. Any change in shape, size or colour, and any bleeding or loss of contour, should be reported to your doctor.

Who is at risk?

We all are. The cumulative effect of the sun is important so people who work outdoors are particularly affected, as are 'tanorexics' – the rays from a sunbed can be ten times that of the midday sun. If you have fair skin and freckles, you are at greater risk, and the same is true if you have more than fifty moles, smoke or have a family history of melanoma.

Preventing it

Eighty per cent of skin cancer is due to ultraviolet rays, so to avoid getting cancer we need to protect against these:

- Stay out of the sun between 11am and 3pm.

Wear clothing and wide-brimmed sunhats and shades to protect the skin.

Wear sunscreen every day of your life. Lots of make-up and moisturisers have SPF 15 in them now.

Use a sunscreen that is water-resistant and sweat-resistant, protects you from ultraviolet A and B and has titanium dioxide as an ingredient. You will need at least two or three tablespoonfuls to apply from top to toe. Don't forget to reapply it every two hours even on a cloudy day as no sunscreen protects 100 per cent and even though sunscreens are water-resistant, they aren't waterproof.

Don't forget your lips.

Buy insect repellant and sun screen separately. You only really need to reapply insect repellant every six to eight hours but sunscreen every couple of hours.

If your sunscreen is smelly or sticky, you won't use it so invest in one you like.

SKIN CANCERS

WHERE MELANOMA OCCURS

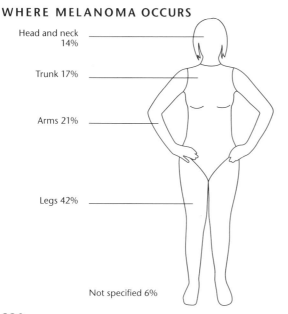

Head and neck 14%

Trunk 17%

Arms 21%

Legs 42%

Not specified 6%

Most of us have heard of malignant melanomas and the dangers of sunbathing. However, although we may be sun-smart, we are often not very skin aware. Non-melanoma skin cancer outnumbers melanoma by nine to one in the UK. Australia has the highest rate of skin cancer, with non-melanoma skin cancers the most common form of cancer. If you reside in Oz and live to be seventy, you have a two in three chance of getting a skin cancer! We tend to spot the more serious form of skin cancer – melanoma – more readily because it occurs in the pigment cells. Unfortunately, non-melanoma cancer occurs in the squamous and basal layers of the skin and is very often missed.

What should I be looking for?

Any spot or sore that hasn't healed after four weeks needs checking, as does any crusty lesion, irregular scaly patch of skin or lump that develops without explanation. Three in every ten cases of non-melanoma cancer occur in those aged under sixty, and 90 per cent are thought to be due to sun damage. We are now seeing more cases and at an increasingly younger age. You are at especially high risk of basal cell carcinoma if you suffered repeated sunburn in childhood.

Spot the difference

A basal cell carcinoma usually occurs on the head and neck and starts as a small, red–pink pearly lump. Basal cell carcinomas occur on the face, hands, ears, scalp, shoulders and back. They can appear shiny, may have blood vessels on the surface and can bleed or become crusty. Although they tend to grow slowly, they form a 'rodent ulcer' if ignored and literally eat away at your face. A squamous cell carcinoma often occurs on the lips, ears, arms, shoulders, face or legs. It starts as a scaly red area that can bulk up and harden.

Things to look out for

A scaly patch of skin that looks like psoriasis may actually be a precancerous area. Crusty lesions on the face, scalp or hands may be precancerous too, so ask your doctor to take a look.

Treatments Many precancerous conditions can be treated by freezing or applying prescription creams. Non-melanoma skin cancers are normally cut out, and you may require radiotherapy to the surrounding tissue afterwards. Potent creams and light therapy are also used. There is an increased risk of further skin cancers if you have already had one removed, so don't think you're off the hook.

Tip ▌ *Gardeners and those who live on the coast are at increased risk – ignore any skin changes at your peril.*

HAIR LOSS

Let's start with simple hair fall – telogen effluvium. The life-cycle of a hair is between ninety and a hundred and twenty days, but this is affected by what goes on inside and outside your head. My teacher Sister Mary John always told me I would make her hair fall out and I just laughed, but it can happen. Stress, illness and childbirth can all result in hair fall about three or four months later. The delay is due to the length of the hair's life-cycle. The good news is that the hair tends to regrow on removal of the stressor.

What about brittle hair?

If your hair is brittle and falling out, look to your diet. Are you taking in enough iron, vitamin B12, zinc, vitamin C, calcium, magnesium and selenium? Are you taking any relevant medicines? Are you inadvertently pulling your hair so it's becoming weak? – ladies who braid their hair often have bald patches at the hair margins. Alternatively, could you have a problem with your thyroid gland? In the meantime, don't wash your hair every day. Gently brush it once a day and avoid tying it up. Boost your iron and vitamin C and B12 to nourish your hair.

What, a receding hairline?

It's not a good look but it's one that unfortunately comes to most of us in time when the menopause hits. Polycystic ovary syndrome and steroids can also cause it. If anything seems different, have your hormones, in particular your testosterone, tested. Minoxidil, which you can get on prescription, will treat it but it needs to be used permanently – if you stop, your hair will recede again.

All about alopecia

It is difficult to estimate how many people suffer, but men and women are equally hit. Alopecia areata is patchy baldness, whereas alopecia totalis occurs when all the body hair is lost, so no lashes, brows, body or pubic hair. This is thankfully less frequent. More than half of all alopecia sufferers are affected before age twenty. A quarter of them have someone in their family who has suffered similarly, and in one in five the nails become pitted.

So what happens here? Just like a person might reject a donor kidney, so your system switches on its antibodies to your own hair. It's a bit like being bitten by your own dog. We call this an autoimmune disease, and these individuals often suffer from other autoimmune diseases, such as thyroid problems, vitamin B12 deficiency and vitiligo – white patches on the skin as the body rejects the cells that make the pigment melanin.

Will my hair grow back? If less than 50 per cent of the hair is affected, there's an 80 per cent chance it will grow back. However, it doesn't bode well if the condition occurs very early in childhood, the nails are affected, there is a family history of autoimmune problems or more than 50 per cent of the scalp is involved.

Can it be treated? Yes, but with limited success. Steroid creams or injections can act as anti-inflammatories and stimulate hair regrowth. Topical tacrolimus, an ointment version of the medicine used to prevent transplant rejections, has also been used to try to stamp it out. DCP is a treatment provided in specialist clinics: a chemical that you have never met before is rubbed into the bald patches in increasing strength to create a reaction. When the skin reacts, this can stimulate the paralysed hair follicles to come to life, with hair regrowth. Some studies cite a 75 per cent success rate, but it doesn't work for everyone.

Wigs Don't baulk at the prospect of a wig – go and get one fitted. If you have some hair remaining, you can have a permanent wig, which is like a mesh weaved into your remaining hair by a specialist hair salon. So ask for a referral, and don't hide under your hat as there is help.

Infectious diseases

13

Find out about what you can catch and importantly, how to get rid of it.

IMPETIGO

A highly contagious infection

A patient once asked me if impetigo had anything to do with impotence; the answer is no, but it has everything to do with a bacterium called *Staphylococcus aureus.* That's a mouthful, but it roughly translates to 'golden cluster seed'. It also translates into a highly infectious condition resulting in pus-filled blisters which burst and leave a patch of inflamed skin that oozes and has a characteristic golden crust.

How do you contract it?

If you come into contact with the *Staphylococcus aureus* bacterium, you may develop impetigo about four to ten days later. In hotter climates, *Streptococcus pyogenes* bacteria are occasionally the culprits, but Staph's usually the big player. It appears as a red sore and then transforms into a yellow crusty lesion, usually around the face, most often the nose and mouth. You catch it from someone with the infection by direct contact with their skin or by using their towels, soap or face cloths. Not surprising then that students, wrestlers and rugby players are prone.

Who gets it?

Impetigo is commonly seen in kids, but because it is so contagious it can spread through a household or student flat like wildfire. The bacterium can gain entry through cracks in the skin caused by skin conditions, or through a graze or insect bite. You can spread it still further by scratching.

Does it go away?

Yes, but it's important to see the doctor for treatment, otherwise you will transfer it to others. Your doctor will know simply by looking at it that it's impetigo. If there's any doubt, a swab can be sent to the lab to confirm the diagnosis by testing for the bacteria.

Treatment is internal and external, so it involves an ointment, usually fusidic acid, and antibiotic tablets, usually flucloxacillin, or erythromycin in those who are allergic to penicillin. The key is to complete the course of antibiotics, which usually lasts seven to ten days. If you wish to remove the crusts, soak a clean cloth in a mixture of half a cup of white vinegar in a litre of tepid water. Place this over the crusts for about ten minutes and then gently wipe them away. Make sure you wash your hands before and after, and bin the cloth as it will harbour germs.

But it's not going away

See the doctor as it is worth checking to see if you are suffering from a chronic Staphylococcus infection. About one in five of the healthy population are chronic carriers of *Staphylococcus aureus,* and it's usually harmless, i.e. they have no infection. You might be one of these people, and this could be why you keep getting infections. So if there is a colony of Staphylococcus growing in your nose and you rub your nose and then touch some cracked skin, you may develop impetigo. Treat it and it will go away, but the colony will remain until you specifically tackle that. Colonies of Staphylococcus can also be found in the groin, the arm pits and the crack between the buttocks – it's got lots of places to hide. The doctor can swab all these areas and check for the culprit. This problem is dealt with by antibiotics, a nasal antibiotic ointment and an antibacterial shower gel, all usually for two weeks.

It's worth bearing in mind that if you suffer from recurrent boils, Staphylococcus carriage may be the cause of this as well.

Other issues

Recurrent infection can occasionally be due to diabetes, low iron, poor nutrition, blood disorders such as lymphomas, alcoholism, intravenous drug abuse, low immunity and kidney problems, so a blood test may be in order if the swabs are negative and the infection keeps cropping up.

Tip *Pick at your peril – this will spread the infection both to you and to others.*

Myth *Impetigo causes scarring. No, it doesn't – it simply disappears without trace on treatment.*

SHINGLES

Shingles infection will strike up on one in four of us in our lifetime. It is due to the reactivation of the chicken pox virus. We call this the varicella zoster virus, and it can lie dormant for decades before it decides to reappear as shingles. It's a bit like a rock band reforming after many years when it sees an opportunity. The quirky name of shingles comes from the Latin word for girdle, which is cingulum, an apt choice as the shingles rash wraps round the body.

How might I catch it?

You don't actually catch shingles; it catches you! It can occur for no apparent reason, but we also see it in those who are stressed and run down, have low immunity or are on certain drugs such as steroids or chemotherapy, which in turn lower their immunity. Shingles can come on after a bout of illness such as a bad bout of flu. Older people also seem to be more susceptible, with the highest risk age group being the over fifties. You generally only get it once, but never say never as about one in fifty people have more than one bout.

Is it like chicken pox?

Ninety per cent of us have chicken pox at some point in our lives, but most of us don't remember it as we were probably only a single-figure age. Shingles differs from chicken pox in that the first symptom tends to be pain. Shingles affects the nerves, so the pain is felt in the skin around the area of the nerve. It can range from a piercing, stabbing pain to a mere tingle. It may also be accompanied by fever and flu-like symptoms. About two to three days after the pain, a rash develops. The rash looks like chicken pox in that it starts as red bumps and these then progress to blisters that eventually scab over. It differs from chicken pox, however, in that it only affects the skin of the surrounding strip of nerve, it never crosses the midline and it doesn't spread. Like the childhood pox, it may be itchy. It is only infectious to those who have not had chicken pox as the blisters of shingles are stuffed with chicken pox virus.

How can I de-shingle myself?

See your doctor as soon as possible to make sure that it is shingles. You may be offered antiviral medication if you see your doctor within seventy-two hours of onset of the rash as this can reduce the severity of the infection.

Is it a big deal, or will I just 'deal' with it?

We call this a 'self-limiting ' infection, which is basically doctor speak for 'it will get better in time on its own'. Medicine doesn't cure it; it simply lessens the symptoms and may have an impact on the complications.

The most common problem is Post Herpetic Neuralgia. This is where you get pain in the site of the rash long after the rash has cleared up. At least 10 per cent of people suffer from this – it can last as little as a month or as long as your lifetime! You are more likely to get this if you are over 50, if you had a severe attack and if you had a lot of pain before the rash arrived. Many treatments are used for this from older antidepressants called amitriptyline, anti-epileptic medicines, to straightforward painkillers. A topical treatment called Capsacin which is made from chillies can also be rubbed onto the area. Don't try and make your own, you can get it on prescription! If you want to go the non-pill route, it is worth trying acupuncture or a TENS machine. (These are used for labour pains, and you can buy your own!)

Problem areas Most shingles occurs on the chest or the back, as a cluster or strip of blisters that then scab over. It can occur anywhere and if it affects the eye prompt action needs to be taken to prevent serious problems as the eye can become scarred by the infection. The blisters themselves can also get infected, so try not to scratch them.

Follow up Check in with your doctor a month after the shingles if you aren't up to scratch. By this stage most of the external signs of the infection will have fled. However it is not uncommon to be left feeling flat and fatigued and lacking your usual fizz. This generally resolves in time.

Pregnant women beware – if you haven't had chicken pox and you come in contact with shingles, you can contract chicken pox from shingles. Shingles sufferers should remain out of circulation until all the lesions have scabbed over. Although it is not as infectious as chicken pox you are still technically contagious.

Oddities

Bizarrely it is possible to be diagnosed with shingles but not have a rash! This uncommon scenario is termed 'Zoster Sine Herpete'. It is also impossible to prevent shingles – if it's in there and it wants to come out, there is no stopping it! Your doctor may mention herpes when they speak to you about shingles. Don't be alarmed. Shingles is one of the family of herpes viruses and contrary to popular opinion, they are not always sexually transmitted.

OH HELL, IT'S HERPES

Genital herpes is caused by one type of the herpes simplex virus. Its incidence in the UK has grown fivefold in the last thirty years, with a peak in the under thirties. It's a sexually transmitted infection, contracted through oral, anal or vaginal sex as well as close contact with other affected areas, such as the eyes and fingers. An infected individual often has no obvious signs signalling you to steer clear.

How would I know I had herpes?

In women, the first attack of genital herpes usually results in a flu-like illness lasting less than a week, and then tingling down below followed by an outbreak of terribly painful blisters and ulcers. Externally, you feel sore, and it hurts to go to the toilet. Your glands often swell, and you may have a low-grade fever. Oddly, these symptoms may not crop up until some time later, maybe when you are run down. The virus then reactivates and gives you symptoms.

Because you can contract herpes from someone without symptoms and pass the infection on to your partner, this can clearly give rise to queries about infidelity. But it's possible for your partner to have signs of herpes without playing away from home. This is because the virus is in their system and has simply become reactivated by illness or stress. Equally, just because you experience a break-out of herpes, this does not mean you have passed it on to your male partner – he could have passed it to you as men very often shed the virus without symptoms, which is why this problem is so rampant.

Will it go away if I ignore it?

No, herpes remains with you for ever. If you don't treat it, you'll probably have symptoms for twenty days. The average person may suffer a further four – generally less painful and shorter – attacks in the next twelve months. Treatment is with antiviral drugs such as aciclovir (acyclovir) or valaciclovir (valacyclovir), ideally as soon as possible. Self-medicating with over-the-counter cold sore ointment (as cold sores are caused by the same virus) won't work, so don't bother. Saline baths help to soothe

the pain, as do painkillers such as ibuprofen and paracetamol. The diagnosis is usually obvious to the doctor, but a swab or blood test can be taken to confirm it if needed.

Recurrent problems?

Don't shy away from the doctor if it keeps coming back. Ask for an emergency supply of aciclovir 200mg tablets. If you take five a day for five days as soon as the symptoms start, you are well on your way to breaking the recurrent cycle. If you are getting more than five bouts a year, ask for suppressive treatment. This involves aciclovir 400mg twice a day for up to a year to quench the herpes fire.

What if I think I've got it?

See your doctor – you'll need a full STI check. Tell your partner; they have often had an episode in the past and either not told you or forgotten about it. A man tends to be more likely to transmit it to a woman than the vice versa, but your partner may have symptoms even if you don't as viral transmission is often silent.

The top priority is to tell your midwife or doctor if you fall pregnant as rarely a genital herpes infection in mum can cause problems for the baby. Blood tests to show if you have been exposed to herpes may take up to twelve weeks to become positive, so an early negative blood test may not be accurate.

Finally, beware the man bearing a cold sore as it too can give rise to genital herpes as it's a herpes simplex virus too. Although type 1 is generally found on the mouth and 2 on the genitals, oral herpes can spread to the genitals or vice versa through oral sex.

CHLAMYDIA – COULD YOU CATCH IT?

As many as one in ten people may carry Chlamydia, and unprotected sex and multiple partners increase your risk. Sadly, symptoms don't often give us a clue because they're absent in 70 per cent of women and over 50 per cent of men. It's no surprise that Chlamydia is catching.

What could the symptoms be?

- Pain when passing urine
- Vaginal discharge
- Bleeding after sex or in between your periods
- Discomfort low down in your tummy.

Beware the man who has pain when having a pee or has any form of discharge from his water pipe. Sadly, though, there is a 50/50 chance a chap carrying Chlamydia won't have any symptoms, so you won't ever know.

How do you catch it?

Unprotected sex is the prime route. Cross-contamination can occur from the hands and mouth, so an unsuspecting sore throat or red eye could be a symptom. Infections in the back passage may cause pain and discharge. Unfortunately, if your partner has been diagnosed with Chlamydia, there's a 66 per cent chance you'll have it too.

What's the big problem?

No symptoms, no diagnosis and as a result no treatment. If left untreated, Chlamydia can result in pelvic inflammatory disease in as many as 40 per cent of cases. So it may only be when it's time to fall pregnant and you fail that you realise you've had Chlamydia. Pelvic inflammatory disease can also increase the risk of ectopic pregnancies or result in an acute pelvic infection requiring admission to hospital.

Tests However you look at it, knowledge of whether you've got it really is power. Chlamydia is tested for by means of an internal swab or sometimes a urine test. If a urine test is used, try not to go the toilet for two hours beforehand.

Good news

Chlamydia is pretty easy to treat. The easiest way is to take a large, one-off dose of an antibiotic called azithromycin. This generally rids the body of Chlamydia, but sex is banned for seven days after the antibiotics and until your partner has been tested and treated.

Who needs to know if I've got it?

If you have symptoms, any partners you have had in the last four weeks need to be informed. If you haven't got any symptoms, you need to go back to all encounters in the last six months. But if you contract Chlamydia from an asymptomatic partner, they may have had it for a long time rather than been unfaithful.

Tip ▎ *Recurrent cystitis may actually be a Chlamydia infection, so have a test.*

Myth ▎ *With every STI comes a symptom. No – this is emphatically not true of Chlamydia, which is more often than not symptom-free.*

HIV

Although there is no cure, HIV is treatable and the vast majority of people living with this disease are doing exactly that and leading normal lives. Those who fare worst are those ignorant of their status. Statistics show that one in four cases would live longer if diagnosed earlier, and a staggering one in seven remain undiagnosed. If in doubt, take a test.

Am I at risk?

Worldwide, over thirty million people are living with HIV. It goes without saying that anyone who has unprotected sex is at risk, so that's a lot of people! Also beware if you pay for sex, engage in bisexual sex or have a bisexual partner, your partner has used prostitutes, especially abroad, or you use intravenous drugs. Blood transfusions and tattoos may pose a risk depending on where they were done.

The number of people with HIV has increased in the last decade, especially in east and central Asia and eastern Europe. In sub-Saharan Africa the rate of HIV infection among adults is stabilising at 5 per cent. But you don't have to go that far for staggering stats – the adult prevalence in the Caribbean is 1.1 per cent and in North America 0.6 per cent, with a global average of 0.8 per cent. We travel a lot, we vaccinate against various infections, we take malaria prophylaxis, yet often we fail to see the hazards of HIV both at home and abroad.

What are the symptoms?

You'll often have few symptoms, but 80 per cent of individuals have a seroconversion reaction two to four weeks after contracting the infection – usually a flu-like illness accompanied by a fever, sore throat and rash. It takes many years to develop AIDS, the ultimate consequence of HIV infection, and treatment delays this progression. HIV makes you prone to diseases that occur with low immunity – colds, diarrhoea, warts, cold sores, tuberculosis, pneumonia.

Testing

You cannot be tested against your will or without prior knowledge and consent. The standard test checks for HIV antibodies in the blood. These can take ninety days to develop, so you can't take a test until this length of time after your encounter. It is now possible to do a combination test at twenty-eight days that checks HIV antibodies and a substance called P24 antigen and allows earlier detection.

Some surgeries do an on the spot fingerprick blood test, which gives a result in ten minutes. This is useful for anxious patients who may be unable to wait several days for their results. It is important to realise that when taking out life insurance, you will not be penalised for having an HIV test, and you only need to disclose information if the test is positive.

Tip *You are at risk if you believe that being gay poses the only risk – there has been a staggering rise in the heterosexual spread of HIV in Western countries.*

Myth *HIV is not transferred though oral sex. It is.*

SYPHILIS

Many women naïvely think of syphilis as occurring in Renaissance times, and indeed it did cause many deaths then. But syphilis is here to stay, and the number of infections is on the up, so it's not to be sniffed at.

What causes it?

The first epidemic in Europe occurred in 1495, and some say that Christopher Columbus brought syphilis back from the New World when he discovered it. No one really knows, but the bottom line is that syphilis – 'the pox' – has been around for years.

It is caused by a bacterium called *Treponema pallidum,* which is transmitted through close bodily contact – skin-to-skin contact or oral, anal or vaginal sex – with someone who is affected. The bacterium causes sores on the skin, and it is acquired through contact with these. These sores may not be visible as they may be internal. Condoms won't completely protect against syphilis, so you could have been exposed in the past.

Who is most likely to contract syphilis?

Men generally succumb more than women, but we are not immune, ladies, and the resurgence of new relationships in newly divorced people who find themselves 'back on the market' has been implicated in the surge. Promiscuity is the biggest risk factor.

What should I be looking for?

Beware the man bearing cuts or sores around his genitalia. Cuts or sores down below that appear to be new or don't heal need checking. (Although they're called sores, they aren't actually sore so don't be fooled.) However, you may see nothing if they're internal. The lesions disappear in a couple of weeks. This stage is called primary syphilis.

Next comes the rash. This appears about three to six weeks after the sores and is often misdiagnosed as eczema or psoriasis. It can occur on the hands and feet or all over the body. This is the most infectious period, and it's sometimes accompanied by fever or flu-like symptoms. There may be patchy hair loss and white patches on the tongue or roof of the mouth. This period of 'secondary' syphilis may last a year, with symptoms coming and going.

245

Then there's a quiet period called latent syphilis, where you show no signs of the disease and cannot spread it. Many years later, if the condition goes undetected, you may develop tertiary syphilis, which can result in damage to the heart, joints, eyes, nervous system and brain. Syphilis can therefore give rise to dementia and paralysis, so it's serious stuff. Just think – the worst effects of your one night stand may not be apparent for twenty years!

Is it treatable?

Yes, that's the annoying thing – if you treat it at the primary stage, it's easy to deal with. Treatment started after then may mean that it has already given rise to problems elsewhere. Treatment is usually by means of a large, painful dose of an antibiotic injection into the backside, but it's worth it!

Be on the look out

See your doctor if you develop any sores around your vagina, vulva or anus, particularly three weeks after a sexual encounter as this is when they start to crop up. And also check in if you develop a rash, or you're treating a rash that isn't going away. If you feel you are at risk, speak up and ask for a syphilis test. It is important to remember that untreated syphilis is not only harmful to you and your partner, but can also result in stillbirth and miscarriage. It is standard practice to screen all pregnant women for syphilis, but don't let this be the occasion you find out you have it. Test for it and fix it as it will not go away on its own. You also need to check for other STIs as well as infections often occur in clusters – you may have Chlamydia or gonorrhoea on the go too.

GONORRHEA

Anecdotally, gonorrhoea has been referred to as 'the clap', from 'les clapiers' meaning rabbit hutches – the name given to brothels in Paris in the Middle Ages. But gonorrhoea is not confined to ladies of the night – it affects all walks of life. And half of all women who have it don't know they do. With the incidence of gonorrhoea going up – it's now number two in the STI charts –this is dangerous. Contrary to what people may think, gonorrhoea is not contracted from toilet seats but through unprotected oral, anal or vaginal sex or the sharing of sex toys.

What might the symptoms be?

Symptoms can crop up one day to two weeks after you come into contact with gonorrhoea. The discharge tends to be thick, smelly and often green. You may bleed between your periods, have pain in your pelvis or experience pain and frequency when passing urine.

Diagnosis It's diagnosed from a swab or a urine test. If you test positive for gonorrhoea, there's a 40 per cent chance you will have Chlamydia too.

Treatment Luckily, it's easily treated with a one-off dose of antibiotic. More strains of gonorrhoea have become resistant to antibiotics, so it's important to make sure your treatment works – you may have to return in seventy-two hours for a further test.

What are the consequences of catching gonorrhoea?

It's possible to develop pelvic inflammatory disease, become infertile or suffer an ectopic pregnancy if this infection goes unchecked. If you think you've got it, get the test and the treatment. Remember that gonorrhoea can crop up in the eyes, anus or throat, so beware a sudden sore throat after an unprotected sexual encounter.

Tip *Ninety per cent of guys with gonorrhoea have symptoms, so look before you leap.*

Myth *Once you catch it, you are immune. Wrong, it's possible to be re-infected, hence the need to treat your partner.*

247

THE ABC OF HEPATITIS

There are several types of hepatitis – inflammation of the liver – but let's stick to the types you might stumble across, the most common contenders being A, B and C.

Hepatitis A

You may have heard of this if you have holidayed in far-flung places as vaccination is often recommended before you travel. Although it commonly occurs where the water isn't pure, it can occur anywhere and is the most common form. It is spread by the faecal-oral route so, put bluntly, if the chef preparing your salad has hepatitis A and wipes his backside but doesn't wash his hands, you may get far more than a salad for lunch.

Hepatitis B and C

Hepatitis B is spread through blood and bodily fluids, so sexual activity, needle sharing and blood transfusion are important. Hepatitis C is transmitted in a similar fashion but tends to be most infectious via the blood. It is classically spread through drug addicts sharing needles.

How bad is hepatitis A?

It's usually a mild infection that passes without significant incident. It may leave you with slightly abnormal liver blood tests, but once it has passed your immunity tends to be lifelong and you make a full recovery.

How bad is hepatitis B?

Hepatitis B is fifty times more infectious than HIV! About two billion people worldwide have been infected with it, and three-quarters of the world's population live in areas where there is a high infection rate. The initial infection will generally come on two to three months after exposure, so a sexual encounter on holiday might not come back to haunt you until next quarter.

Only half of those affected get jaundice – go yellow – so people often just stay home feeling like they have flu. Other symptoms are pain below the right rib cage, sometimes fever, feeling run down, a sickly sensation and loss of appetite. It can last up to six weeks, but most healthy people recover. It can occasionally be severe and rarely result in liver failure and death.

About one in twenty patients never clear the virus, which leads to chronic hepatitis B infection. This can lead to cirrhosis of the liver and liver cancer – a horrible death.

How bad is hepatitis C?

This disease is a big problem as it may be lifelong in 75 per cent of individuals. It may give symptoms of tiredness and flu, put you off your food, give you jaundice and make you intolerant of alcohol, but often has no symptoms. If so, you have no idea you have it until complications start to set in. Long-term infection with hepatitis C can result in cirrhosis, liver cancer and ultimately death.

What would put me at risk of hepatitis?

Unprotected sex is a gamble; don't go there. And about 50 per cent of intravenous drug users in large capital cities carry hepatitis C. Don't have tattoos or medical or dental treatment abroad unless it's an emergency as you could be at risk of B and C.

If you are partial to a rolled-up note of cocaine, bear in mind that, as well as seriously damaging your health, you could catch hepatitis B or C. Healthcare workers, police officers and prison staff are at risk of blood-borne hepatitis.

Vaccination

We can vaccinate against hepatitis A and B but not C. Hepatitis A vaccine involves one shot and a booster one year later to confer twenty years' immunity. Hepatitis B vaccination involves three shots – at day one, and one and six months. You should periodically check your immune status via a blood test, especially if you are a healthcare worker, and boosters may be needed every five years. The vaccination may be ineffective if you are overweight.

The price of paradise

Always check your immunisation schedule when heading abroad – the price you pay for contracting hepatitis is far greater than the price of the inoculation or your holiday. Think hepatitis if you become ill on return from a foreign holiday, and ask for a test.

Diet and metabolism

14

You are what you eat – here are some handy tips on how to fill in your nutritional gaps.

DIABETES

Diabetes is one of the top killers. It's estimated that the number of people with diabetes will double in the next twenty-five years, and in the UK, we're already spending 10 per cent of our healthcare budget on it. About one in thirty people in the UK are currently aware that they suffer from diabetes.

But I feel fine so I must be fine!

Wrong! There are an estimated 750,000 people living with diabetes in the UK who are blissfully unaware of it. Just because you did not develop diabetes as a child or an adolescent doesn't mean you're safe. Type 2 diabetes tends to come on in adulthood and often goes unnoticed.

What are the symptoms?

People tend to feel thirsty and tired, want to pass urine frequently and sometimes lose weight. Recurrent infections like thrush, boils or cystitis may occur. Occasionally the diagnosis is simply picked up incidentally.

INCREASED RISK OF DIABETES

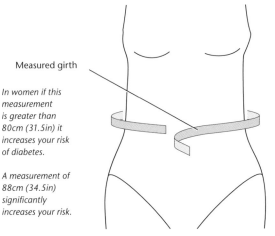

Measured girth

In women if this measurement is greater than 80cm (31.5in) it increases your risk of diabetes.

A measurement of 88cm (34.5in) significantly increases your risk.

How is it tested for?

If your doctor thinks you may have diabetes, you will need to have blood and urine tests. Any sugar in your urine is the first clue. A fasting blood sugar level will give you your score on the day – ideally this should fall below 6mmol/l (126mg/dl). An HbA1c can be done to provide a guide to your average blood sugar over the last few months. A glucose tolerance test can be carried out too – blood sugar level is recorded and then you're given a blood sugar load and your blood is retested at intervals. This is frequently carried out in pregnant

251

women who are deemed to be at risk – if they have a parent with diabetes, are overweight or have given birth to a large baby.

What causes diabetes?

Insulin is needed to break down blood sugar; we can't live without it. People with type 1 diabetes have to have insulin injections as they don't have insulin. In type 2 diabetes, either we don't make enough insulin or our body doesn't react to it. So our blood glucose becomes high and causes symptoms.

Who is at risk?

Eighty per cent of people with type 2 diabetes are overweight. As a woman, you have an increased risk if you have a waist size of 80cm (31.5in) or greater. Afro-Caribbean and South Asian women, those who are over forty, and ladies who developed diabetes in pregnancy are also more prone.

Complications

High blood sugar can cause havoc – kidney disease, blindness, problems with circulation and bladder and bowel control, strokes, heart attacks. One thing's for sure, it will lead to problems, and the longer it goes unchecked, the worse these are.

Treatment The good news is that this disease can often be managed with diet alone. Tablets are sometimes needed, and very rarely insulin. The aim of the game is to keep the sugar low and prevent any complications of diabetes. Rigorous checks are made on blood pressure, cholesterol and kidneys. Eyes, skin, feet and circulation are assessed on a regular basis. You may feel fine, but diabetes never goes away.

Tips
- *Have the flu and pneumonia vaccinations – diabetes impairs the immune response so if there's anything going round, you're far more likely to catch it.*
- *Get your vitamin B12 levels checked as these are often low if you have diabetes.*
- *Learn about your disease and let people know you have it.*

Myths
- *Remember there's no such thing as a 'touch' of diabetes – you either have it or you don't.*
- *Diabetes is due to eating too many sweet things. No, it's not really what you eat but how much you eat that counts as weight is the determining factor.*

OBESITY

No one likes to be called obese; it's a horrid word that conjures up horrid images. Worse still is 'morbidly obese' – that's the worse insult ever. The latter is when your BMI, short for body mass index, hits 40. You can calculate this by dividing your weight by your height squared. Ideally, your BMI should fall between 20 and 25. Have a look at the chart on page 255 – how do you fare?

The other hot topic in terms of weight is abdominal girth. That's simply how you measure up around your abdomen, at your belly button. Girls whose girth is greater than 80cm (31.5in) substantially increase their risk of developing diabetes later in life. So get the measuring tape out. If you are coming up high, ask yourself the following questions:

- Do I skip breakfast?
- Do I eat three meals a day?
- Do I snack, and if so, on what?
- Do I drink one to two litres (two or three pints) of water a day?
- Do I buy ready meals and takeaways?
- How much exercise am I taking?
- Do I ever have 'seconds', and do I only eat off a plate?

Simply put, ladies, it's a supply and demand issue here. Your system needs to burn off any high-fat, high-sugar you load it up with. If you indulge, you must burn it off. Some of us do this more efficiently than others, but some of us also eat more than others.

Is it a problem with my glands doctor?

Countless women have sat in my surgery hoping that their weight gain was due to a thyroid problem, but it usually isn't. There are, however, basic tests that you need to have, including on your thyroid gland, for diabetes, for liver and kidney function and very importantly your cholesterol level.

What about diet pills?

Orlistat has an effect on the absorption of fat into the bloodstream so that any fat you eat, you'll effectively excrete. That sounds straightforward, but if you don't limit your fat intake, you'll end up with offensive orange diarrhoea, which is very unpleasant. Orlistat stops the absorption of one third of the fat you take in and excretes it. It's possible to lose 10 per cent of your body weight within six months. The drug is available over the counter in some countries, including the UK and Australia, but the standard therapeutic dose of 120mg taken three times a day is available only on prescription. It is best advised for those with a BMI of over 30 or a BMI of 28 and a medical condition such as diabetes.

What about surgery?

Obesity surgery Diet and exercise are the key tools to weight loss, but many women fail to achieve their goal. We all have a friend who eats like a horse yet is a slim as a whippet, and similarly some of us are destined to carry more weight than others. Many patients don't contemplate surgery because they fear it, feel that it's a cheat or genuinely hope that there is a quick-fix drug or diet that can help. Often there isn't, and bearing in mind the long-term health risks of obesity, surgery can make sense.

Gastric band This is procedure whereby a band is placed at the top of the stomach, creating an upper pocket about the size of a plum. When this fills, food is released into the lower part of the stomach, the idea being that you feel fuller faster and for longer. The procedure is done under general anaesthetic using keyhole surgery and normally takes less than an hour. You will usually be left with some small cuts on your abdomen where the surgeon has entered with the telescopic camera. The band is secured tightly around the stomach so you don't have to worry about its coming undone! It can be tightened or loosened by means of an access port hidden below your ribs. The beauty of it is that it is both reversible and adjustable, meaning that you can control your stomach capacity.

Who is a candidate for banding? Anyone whose BMI is 40 or over, and anyone with a BMI of 35 or over with obesity-related complications, for example diabetes.

BODY MASS INDEX

Use this chart to find your body mass index. Ideally, your BMI should fall between 20 and 25.

Weight in kilograms

Height in centimetres

kg	142	145	147	150	152	155	158	160	163	165	168	170	173	175	178	180	183	Weight in stones and pounds
40	20	19	19	18	17	17	16	16	15	15	14	14	13	13	13	12	12	6st 4
41	20	20	19	18	18	17	16	16	15	15	15	14	14	13	13	13	12	6st 6
42	21	20	19	19	18	17	17	16	16	15	15	15	14	14	13	13	13	6st 9
43	21	20	20	19	19	18	17	17	16	16	15	15	14	14	14	13	13	6st 11
44	22	21	20	20	19	18	18	17	17	16	16	15	15	14	14	14	13	6st 13
45	22	21	21	20	19	19	18	18	17	17	16	16	15	15	14	14	13	7st 1
46	23	22	21	20	20	19	18	18	17	17	16	16	15	15	15	14	14	7st 3
47	23	22	22	21	20	20	19	18	18	17	17	16	16	15	15	15	14	7st 6
48	24	23	22	21	21	20	19	19	18	18	17	17	16	16	15	15	14	7st 8
49	24	23	23	22	21	20	20	19	18	18	17	17	16	16	15	15	15	7st 10
50	25	24	23	22	22	21	20	20	19	18	18	17	17	16	16	15	15	7st 12
51	25	24	24	23	22	21	20	20	19	19	18	18	17	17	16	16	15	8st
52	26	25	24	23	23	22	21	20	20	19	18	18	17	17	16	16	16	8st 3
53	26	25	25	24	23	22	21	21	20	19	19	19	18	17	17	16	16	8st 5
54	27	26	25	24	23	22	22	21	20	20	19	19	18	18	17	17	16	8st 7
55	27	26	25	24	24	23	22	21	21	20	19	19	18	18	17	17	16	8st 9
56	28	27	26	25	24	23	22	22	21	21	20	19	19	18	18	17	17	8st 11
57	28	27	26	25	25	24	23	22	21	21	20	20	19	19	18	18	17	9st
58	29	28	27	26	25	24	23	23	22	21	21	20	19	19	18	18	17	9st 2
59	29	28	27	26	26	25	24	23	22	22	21	20	20	19	19	18	18	9st 4
60	30	29	28	27	26	25	24	23	23	22	21	21	20	20	19	19	18	9st 6
61	30	29	28	27	26	25	24	24	23	22	22	21	20	20	19	19	18	9st 9
62	31	29	29	28	27	26	25	24	23	23	22	21	21	20	20	19	19	9st 11
63	31	30	29	28	27	26	25	25	24	23	22	22	21	21	20	19	19	9st 13
64	32	30	30	28	28	27	26	25	24	24	23	22	21	21	20	20	19	10st 1
65	32	31	30	29	28	27	26	25	24	24	23	22	22	21	21	20	19	10st 3
66	33	31	31	29	29	27	26	26	25	24	23	23	22	22	21	20	20	10st 6
67	33	32	31	30	29	28	27	26	25	25	24	23	22	22	21	21	20	10st 8
68	34	32	31	30	29	28	27	27	26	25	24	24	23	22	21	21	20	10st 10
69	34	33	32	31	30	29	28	27	26	25	24	24	23	23	22	21	21	10st 12
70	35	33	32	31	30	29	28	27	26	26	25	24	23	23	22	22	21	11st
71	35	34	33	32	31	30	28	28	27	26	25	25	24	23	22	22	21	11st 3
72	36	34	33	32	31	30	29	28	27	26	26	25	24	24	23	22	21	11st 5
73	36	35	34	32	32	30	29	29	27	27	26	25	24	24	23	23	22	11st 7
74	37	35	34	33	32	31	30	29	28	27	26	26	25	24	23	23	22	11st 9
75	37	36	35	33	32	31	30	29	28	28	27	26	25	24	24	23	22	11st 11
76	38	36	35	34	33	32	30	30	29	28	27	26	25	25	24	23	23	12st
77	38	37	36	34	33	32	31	30	29	28	27	27	26	25	24	24	23	12st 2
78	39	37	36	35	34	32	31	30	29	29	28	27	26	25	25	24	23	12st 4
79	39	38	37	35	34	33	32	31	30	29	28	27	26	26	25	24	24	12st 6
80	40	38	37	36	35	33	32	31	30	29	28	27	26	26	25	25	24	12st 8
81	40	39	37	36	35	34	32	32	30	30	29	28	27	26	26	25	24	12st 11
82	41	39	38	36	35	34	33	32	31	30	29	28	27	27	26	25	24	12st 13
83	41	39	38	37	36	35	33	32	31	30	29	29	28	27	26	26	25	13st 1
84	42	40	39	37	36	35	34	33	32	31	30	29	28	27	27	26	25	13st 3
85	42	40	39	38	37	35	34	33	32	31	30	29	28	28	27	26	25	13st 5
86	43	41	40	38	37	36	34	34	32	32	30	30	29	28	27	27	26	13st 8
87	43	41	40	39	38	36	35	34	33	32	31	30	29	28	27	27	26	13st 10
88	44	42	41	39	38	37	35	34	33	32	31	30	29	29	28	27	26	13st 12
89	44	42	41	40	39	37	36	35	33	33	32	31	30	29	28	27	27	14st
90	45	43	42	40	39	37	36	35	34	33	32	31	30	29	28	28	27	14st 2
	4ft 8	4ft 9	4ft 10	4ft 11	5ft 0	5ft 1	5ft 2	5ft 3	5ft 4	5ft 5	5ft 6	5ft 7	5ft 8	5ft 9	5ft 10	5ft 11	6ft	

Height in feet and inches

Imperial measures given are only approximates.

Results On average, people lose 50 per cent of their weight within two years of their gastric band. But although the gastric band will help you lose weight, you're still in total control of what you put into your mouth. For the first four weeks, you will be limited to puréed food and four small meals a day. By week six, you should be eating three meals a day of solid food, i.e. back to your normal eating patterns. Remember to stop eating as soon as you feel full, and avoid drinking at mealtimes as it speeds up the passage of food. Aim to drink a litre or two of water a day.

Pitfalls ▌ *Remember that you'll need to avoid returning to bad eating habits.*

Perks ▌ *If you wish, you can have your gastric band removed and your stomach will revert to its normal size.*

LACK OF IRON

Iron deficiency is the most common nutritional deficiency worldwide. The medical terminology for the condition associated with this is anaemia. It's commonly seen in women due to lack of iron in the diet or increased loss from menstrual cycle. We need more iron on a daily basis than men, and we become particularly demanding of our iron sources around pregnancy and menstruation.

What's so important about iron?

Iron is one of the building blocks of our red blood cells, so it's vital as these are the transport vehicles that carry oxygen around our bodies. Decrease the iron and the transport system slows down, meaning oxygen will not be able to travel round very efficiently.

Symptoms

Tiredness is one of the main symptoms. You can also feel short of breath, feel cold or suffer from palpitations, dizziness or headache. Concentration can be impaired or you might start feeling cranky. Tinnitus can sometimes be a symptom.

What signs might the doctor look for?

You need iron for healthy skin, hair and nails. Hair can become brittle and fall out easily, and nails become crumbly. You mouth might suffer too, with ulcers, cracks around the side and a sore tongue. When your doctor feels your pulse, it might be fast, and you may even have a soft heart murmur. You hands may feel cold and your complexion look ghostly pale.

Who is at risk?

If your periods are excessively heavy, you may succumb. Vegetarians and vegans can also suffer due to inadequate dietary intake. Anyone who suffers from coeliac disease (from an inability to digest gluten) or has other bowel disorders, such as Crohn's disease or ulcerative colitis, is also potentially at risk.

Could there be other reasons?

Yes, and this is the important bit. Although ladies have periods, pregnancy and diet as reasons for developing anaemia, it's vital to get checked if none of these seems applicable to you. A low iron level can sometimes be due to a bleeding ulcer or a bowel cancer, or the first sign of a disease such as coeliac disease. Don't get me wrong, this is usually not the case, but anaemia in any woman over fifty definitely warrants further testing. This usually takes the form of an upper and lower bowel telescopic examination to rule out ulcers, cancer and inflammation.

What are the basic tests?

You will need to have a blood test called a full blood count – this checks your haemoglobin level, which is effectively your cash flow in terms of iron currency. You should also have your ferritin levels checked as these reflect your iron stores, i.e. how much iron you have in the bank. You may have a normal haemoglobin level but a low level of ferritin, meaning that when your iron demand is high you don't have enough on deposit to cater for it. It's a bit like going on a big spend and exceeding your overdraft limit. Iron deficiency classically shows up as small, pale red blood cells on your blood film.

Your doctor may want to do other tests, for example to examine the bowel motions or do a urine test to check for blood. The doctor is likely to do other basic tests, such as for diabetes and thyroid function if you are tired, and in addition check your levels of vitamin B12 and folic acid, both of which are involved in making red blood cells so can contribute to anaemia.

What's next?

You are going to need to boost your diet with iron-rich foods (see Supplements at the end of this section). You will also need to take iron supplements to push your levels up and improve your stores. Iron tablets are not very palatable and often give rise to tummy pain, constipation and diarrhoea. They will also turn your stools black. The dosage is normally two or three tablets per day.

Vitamin C is vital for the absorption of iron so is a must in your diet as well. Imagine iron as your credit card and vitamin C as its PIN number – one is useless without the other. Take your iron supplements with a glass of freshly squeezed orange juice and also drink one with every meal to help absorb as much iron as possible per sitting. It's possible to get tablets that combine iron and vitamin C to aid absorption.

Progress

Further blood tests a few months down the line will tell you how your body is reacting. Treatment usually involves identifying the cause, and as that is commonly diet related it generally improves within two months of supplements. The key thing is to keep the levels topped up by an adequate dietary intake.

Tip *If your offer to donate blood has been declined because your iron count is too low, see your doctor for further tests.*

THYROID PROBLEMS

Thyroid problems are relatively common. The thyroid gland sits just below the Adam's apple and produces a hormone called thyroxine (T4). The gland sets the pace for our metabolism – if it slows down, we slow down and vice versa. So it's not surprising the symptoms can be very varied, and it's a diagnosis that is often missed.

Thyroid blood test results can be confusing, so here's an idiot's guide! Imagine your thyroid is like an open fire and the flame it's emitting is your thyroid function, corresponding to the level of T4 on your lab test. In order to keep the fire burning we need to add kindle – a lot if the flame is low, a little if it's raging. The kindle is the equivalent of the lab test result for thyroid-stimulating hormone – TSH. So we have higher levels if the thyroid gland is slow. And this is where people get confused – a slow thyroid will show up as a low T4 but a high TSH. And an overactive thyroid will show the opposite. Occasionally T4 levels may be normal but TSH too high or too low, indicating that the thyroid may be becoming overstretched or slowing down.

Symptoms of a slow, underactive gland include tiredness, weight gain, constipation, dryness or even loss of the hair, dry skin, irregular periods, weakness/dizzy spells and low mood. It's really simple to diagnose – the doctor will take a blood test for thyroid function. An underactive thyroid gland usually means you need to take treatment for life as your gland is unlikely to start producing enough T4. It seems awful to be told this but think of T4 as being a supplement. Remember it's vital not to stop taking it just because you feel fine as you will again end up with a 'go slow'. In the UK, patients who have thyroid problems are entitled to free National Health Service prescriptions for life, even if they're not related to the thyroid problem.

How likely am I to have an underactive thyroid?

We call this hypothyroidism. Believe me, many women present to the doctor with symptoms of tiredness and weight gain and hope they have a thyroid problem! The reality is that about one in fifty of us are susceptible, whereas only one in a thousand men are. We also see it in the year after pregnancy, and this is when it gets missed as doctors often tell you it's normal to be overweight, tired, irritable and constipated after a baby. So bear this in mind.

The most common reason for a slow thyroid gland is autoimmune thyroiditis. This means your immune response is triggered to reject your thyroid gland. It's a bit like your dog biting you as it no longer recognises you as its owner. It's most common in women aged between twenty and forty and usually causes swelling of the neck – a goitre. If you have a family history of other types of autoimmune disease, such as vitiligo or pernicious anaemia, or if you suffer from these conditions, you are more likely to be affected.

In some areas of the world, iodine is deficient in the diet, and this causes the thyroid to be underactive as iodine plays an integral part in making thyroid hormone. About one billion people worldwide are affected by iodine deficiency, especially in Latin America and the Caribbean. It's far less likely in Europe, America and Australia due to the availability of iodised salt in supermarkets – adding the supplement into salt has made great inroads into this deficiency. Some medicines can cause an underactive thyroid gland, for example lithium, used in bipolar depression, and amiodarone, used to treat abnormal heart rhythms.

What about an overactive thyroid?

This is less common than underactive thyroid. It's also more difficult to treat. Whereas an underactive gland slows down bodily functions, an overactive one speeds everything up. Symptoms include tremor, irritability, sweating, thinning or loss of the hair, diarrhoea, heavy periods, weight loss yet a big appetite, feeling like a nervous wreck, itchiness and eye problems. In this case, the person sitting before the doctor is usually slim, full of nervous energy, eyeballs protruding and gaunt looking. The condition occurs in about two in one hundred women and two in one thousand men.

Treatment Your family doctor can easily treat an underactive thyroid gland. You will be given T4 supplements, altering the dose on the basis of your blood levels. Once established on it, you usually remain on it for life.

An overactive thyroid is usually treated by a specialist as it requires close monitoring. Normally, a tablet called carbimazole is given to slow the gland. This generally takes about two years of treatment and requires regular blood tests. Other options include radioactive iodine treatment, which nukes the thyroid gland and slows it down, but this isn't suitable for everyone.

Tired all the time?

Get a test – it could be your thyroid talking. Just because you have one normal thyroid test doesn't mean it's normal for ever, so go back if your symptoms are bothering you.

VITAMIN B12 DEFICIENCY

Vitamin B12 is my favourite vitamin! Its main source is meat, fish, eggs and dairy products and if we eat a balanced diet, we are not at risk of deficiency. But, as many of us know, it's really difficult to stick to a healthy eating plan. Vegans are highly at risk of B12 deficiency.

How would I know if I had a deficiency?

You'll feel run down. Your tongue may become sore and the sides of your mouth cracked. Sometimes you'll experience pins and needles, muscular aches and pains, dizziness and headaches. Your friends might comment that you are pale or a lemon colour, and your hair and nails may become cracked and weak. You may be more prone to infections. Some people even become colour blind. Also, your feet may feel funny, with the sensation of pins and needles, often described as walking on cotton wool.

Why do I need vitamin B12?

Vitamin B12 is vital for the production of red blood cells, the vehicles that carry oxygen around the body. Without B12, the red blood cells don't divide, so you are left with fat red blood cells. If you equate these to larger people racing around a track, it's no surprise they are inefficient, and the lack of B12 gives symptoms of anaemia. A long-term lack of vitamin B12 also affects the nerves, resulting in loss of sensation in the hands and feet and, in severe cases, poor concentration, depression and even dementia.

I eat meat so I can't be at risk, right?

If you adhere to a healthy balanced diet, you're likely to be OK. But we only absorb dietary vitamin B12 if we have a substance called intrinsic factor. This is a bit like the 'X factor' in B12 terms. Some people develop antibodies against intrinsic factor, so B12 in the diet gets excreted instead of stored. This condition is called pernicious anaemia and is the most common cause of vitamin B12 deficiency in the UK. Other conditions that make vitamin B12 deficiency more likely are diabetes and bowel disorders such as coeliac disease and Crohn's disease. Patients who have had stomach surgery can also be at risk, and some epilepsy medicines lower levels of B12.

So what do I do?

If you have a family history of pernicious anaemia, you should have a test. The condition is more common in women and those with other autoimmune problems. It's important to diagnose it, both to help your symptoms and because you are three times more likely to develop stomach cancer. If your B12 levels are low, you will automatically have a blood test for intrinsic factor antibodies. The condition is treated by B12 injections.

Vegan?

If you are a strict vegetarian, a vegan or have a poor diet, you may be B12 deficient. You can take B12 supplements by mouth. If it's very severe, you may need an injection as this boosts levels within forty-eight hours whereas a supplement may take four to six weeks for the same effect.

SUPPLEMENTS

Why do we bother with vitamins and supplements? Our grandmothers never did. That's probably because what they ate would now reside exclusively in the expensive, organic aisle of a supermarket. It was not uncommon to eat in the afternoon what was in the soil in the morning, so supplements weren't needed. But now is a time of pesticides, microwave meals, stress, road rage, and mobile-phone addiction to mention but a few of our vices. We lead different lives and we simply haven't the time or resources to live like granny did, so we need a helping hand. There really is a pill for every ill, but some are more important than others. Here is my guide to the must-have vitamins and minerals.

Calcium

This is the building block of bones. You can get it from dairy products, but if for some reason you can't have them, you can get it through cereals, kale or broccoli. We use 1 per cent of our calcium for hormones and for nerve and muscle function, storing the remainder in our bones. Our bones are constantly remodelling, and as this slows down in menopause along with the absorption of calcium, we often need to top it up. This is vital to prevent osteoporosis, i.e. porous bones which fracture easily.

If you aren't having periods from stress, illness or excessive exercise, you should think about your calcium. Certain medication, for example antiepileptics, can affect calcium metabolism, so again you might need to chew on supplements. Ladies who drink excessive amounts of caffeine or alcohol can have difficulty absorbing calcium. Eating calcium is a bit like eating chalk, and you will often get a fizzy sensation in your belly causing cramps, bloatedness and sometimes wind, so be warned!

Iron

Iron deficiency is the most common deficiency worldwide. Women who have heavy periods, are pregnant or have a chronic illness have a greater demand for iron. We primarily need it to make haemoglobin, the 'taxi' that carries oxygen round the body. If there isn't enough iron, there will be symptoms of lethargy and tiredness.

263

You can get iron in two ways – diet or supplementation. It's found in red meat, fortified cereals, white beans, lentils, spinach, even bread. If you take iron supplements, start at half the recommended daily dose for the first few days to limit the side-effects of diarrhoea, constipation, nausea, vomiting and abdominal pain. Taking iron with vitamin C helps absorption, so swallow it with some fresh orange juice. Be warned though, your bowel motions will start to look a bit black when you take iron supplements. If you drink lots of tea, take care as it contains tannins – the things that stain your teeth – which interfere with iron absorption.

Zinc

Remember this one from chemistry class? Well, it helps with our immunity, which is probably why it can be found in cold and flu remedies. It's also needed for growth and development, wound healing, chemical reactions and bizarrely our sense of taste and smell. Our systems don't have any storage space for zinc, so we need to take it in daily. Oysters contain more zinc than any other food, but beef, cereals, crab, cashews, beans and cheese have high levels too.

Lack of zinc could result in hair loss, lack of concentration, taste problems, delayed healing of wounds, recurrent infections and diarrhoea. Those who are breastfeeding, are alcohol dependent or have sickle cell disease are more likely to be deficient. It's not offered as a standard blood test but can be tested for if, for example, you have unexplained hair loss or taste disruption.

An intake of excessive zinc supplements can have a toxic effect – you'd probably need to eat a minimum of fifteen oysters every day to develop toxicity. My feeling is that cereals are the best way to source zinc on a daily basis, and far cheaper than oysters.

Magnesium

This is another distant memory from chemistry class. It has over three hundred functions in the body. It helps to keep the heart beating, the immune system functioning and the nerves, muscles and bones healthy. Green vegetables, nuts and water all contain it, and the harder your tap water, the greater the magnesium level. We don't often see magnesium deficiency, which presents as nausea, vomiting, fatigue and weakness. It's more often the result of another condition, such as kidney problems, than a lack of magnesium in the diet. If you have Crohn's disease, take water tablets or are an alcoholic, you could need supplements. They are also thought to help with premenstrual syndrome and migraine. However, if the rest of us stick to our five a day and our water drinking, we should be fine.

Vitamin A

This vitamin helps us to see, grow, fight off infections and reproduce. It comes from whole milk, liver and fortified products such as cereals, as well as some fruit and veg – yes, carrots. We don't often see vitamin A deficiency in the UK, but it can occur in countries whose inhabitants are malnourished. Night blindness is the first sign of deficiency. Supplements may be needed in those who do not absorb vitamin A because of gut illnesses, for example coeliac or Crohn's disease. The average person is unlikely to be deficient though, and eating liver once a week will boost your stores of both vitamin A and iron. Daily cereals are again the way to go if you hate liver and carrots.

Team vitamin B

Vitamin B6 is used for lots of chemical reactions in the body – in the function of nerves, muscles and the immune system and the making of red blood cells. Cereals, beans, potatoes, poultry and some fruit and veg contain it. In a developed country, it's rare to be deficient in it – signs include tiredness, a sore tongue, depression and nerve problems.

Should I be supplementing vitamin B? Alcoholics are the most vulnerable when it comes to low B6 levels, with malnourished elderly patients not far behind. The average person is unlikely to lack it, but there is anecdotal evidence that it helps in premenstrual syndrome, so supplementing it when it's your time of the month may help. But take care – B6 overdose can result in nerve damage.

Vitamin B12 is needed to keep nerves and red blood cells healthy. It's found in poultry, fish, meat and milk but not fruit and vegetables, so vegans and vegetarians may need to rely on fortified cereals. If you lack it (see page 261), you can become irritable and run down, and develop constipation, loss of appetite and pins and needles. You can become depressed, confused or even demented, so, girls, this is a serious one. People who have pernicious anaemia cannot absorb vitamin B12 and need it topped up through a minimum of quarterly vitamin B12 injections.

Vitamin D

When the sun is out, the body produces vitamin D, but very few foods provide it. We can source it from fish, in particular tuna meat or cod liver oil – yuk, I hear you say! It's also added to orange juice, cereal and milk. Its prime function is in the absorption of calcium to build up the bones and mineralise the teeth. This is why it's often taken with calcium supplementation.

Vitamin D is in the news a lot as there are estimates that as many as one in three of us are running low in it and as many as 20 per cent of us could be deficient in it. The elderly are particularily at risk and those who rarely see the sun. Pregnant women and patients with Crohn's disease suffer. Not only is it linked to osteoporosis, it also has an association with chronic fatigue, muscular aches and pains, irritability, depression, and our old friend, the symptom of feeling 'tired all the time'. So this might be one to supplement, especially in winter.

Be aware, however, that too much vitamin D can make you feel sick and weak, lose your appetite and lose weight. Taken with calcium, it can increase your risk of kidney stones. Excessive sunlight or a diet rich in vitamin D rarely cause you to build up excessive amounts of vitamin D – as a rule, toxicity results from excessive supplementation. Your doctor can do a blood test to check your vitamin D levels.

Vitamin E

We know this one because it's supposed to help scar tissue. It's also an antioxidant, meaning that it serves as a vacuum cleaner to mop up substances called free radicals – in cigarette smoke, etc. – that can damage cells. Nuts, even peanut butter, seeds such as sunflower seeds, and kiwis, mangos and vegetable oil all contain it. Deficiency is rare. Those who have had coronary heart disease often take supplements as it may prevent or delay coronary heart disease. It is sometimes used in eye clinics to help age-related eye disease and prevent blindness.

Excessive amounts in the diet do not seem to cause problems. But excessive supplementation can sometimes cause a problem with blood clotting and result in haemorrhage. Because of this, supplements should not be taken in patients on warfarin – warfarin is used to prevent the blood clotting and is often taken by people with heart complaints and those who have had blood clots. It's closely monitored so most people will be well versed in telling the pharmacist they're taking it.

Vitamin K

We find this stuff in our greens, olive oil and soya beans. We also grow it in our gut. Deficiency is rare but this can occur with liver disease or blood disorders. It's always tested for if you have a problem with blood clotting. Vitamin K deficiency tends to be the domain of newborn babies as they don't get a lot of it through the placenta, so they're at risk of bleeding – this is why they're given vitamin K after birth. But adults shouldn't really need to supplement it.

The bottom line

Take as many supplements and tonics as you like, but the best route to becoming bionic is to eat your five fruit and veg a day, exercise, drink one or two litres (two to four pints) of water a day and de-stress. Contentment is a tonic in itself!